COMPLEXITY OF THE SELF

THE GUILFORD CLINICAL PSYCHOLOGY AND
PSYCHOTHERAPY SERIES
Michael J. Mahoney, *Editor*

COMPLEXITY OF THE SELF: A DEVELOPMENTAL
APPROACH TO PSYCHOPATHOLOGY AND THERAPY
Vittorio F. Guidano

EMOTION IN PSYCHOTHERAPY: AFFECT, COGNITION, AND THE
PROCESS OF CHANGE
Leslie S. Greenberg and Jeremy D. Safran

RELAPSE PREVENTION: MAINTENANCE STRATEGIES IN THE
TREATMENT OF ADDICTIVE BEHAVIORS
G. Alan Marlatt and Judith R. Gordon, *Editors*

COGNITIVE–BEHAVIORAL THERAPY FOR IMPULSIVE CHILDREN
Philip C. Kendall and Lauren Braswell

PAIN AND BEHAVIORAL MEDICINE: A COGNITIVE–BEHAVIORAL
PERSPECTIVE
Dennis C. Turk, Donald Meichenbaum, and Myles Genest

COGNITIVE PROCESSES AND EMOTIONAL DISORDERS:
A STRUCTURAL APPROACH TO PSYCHOTHERAPY
V. F. Guidano and G. Liotti

AGORAPHOBIA: NATURE AND TREATMENT
Andrew M. Mathews, Michael G. Gelder, and Derek W. Johnston

COGNITIVE ASSESSMENT
Thomas V. Merluzzi, Carol R. Glass, and Myles Genest, *Editors*

COGNITIVE THERAPY OF DEPRESSION
Aaron T. Beck, A. John Rush, Brian F. Shaw, and Gary Emery

COMPLEXITY OF THE SELF
A DEVELOPMENTAL APPROACH TO PSYCHOPATHOLOGY AND THERAPY

VITTORIO F. GUIDANO
Center for Cognitive Therapy
Rome, Italy

THE GUILFORD PRESS
New York   London

Library of Congress Cataloging-in-Publication Data

Guidano, V. F.
  Complexity of the self

  (The Guilford clinical pyschology and psychotherapy series)
  Bibliography: p.
  Includes index.
  1. Self. 2. Psychology, Pathological.
3. Developmental psychology. I. Title. II. Series.
[DNLM: 1. Cognition Disorders. 2. Ego. 3. Mental Disorders—etiology. 4. Mental
Disorders—therapy. 5. Self concept. WM 100 G946c]
RC455.4.S42G85   1987   616.89   87-350
ISBN 0-89862-012-0

To Mike Mahoney and to the timeless time of our conversations in Piazza Navona and Le Papillon.

ACKNOWLEDGMENTS

I wish to acknowledge my gratitude to the Center for Cognitive Therapy of Rome for their assistance and cooperation, and in particular to my friends Mario Reda and Antonio Caridi, with whom I have long and fruitfully discussed the principal ideas presented in this book. I also thank Priscilla De Angelis and William Lyddon for helping me put the work in the final English form.

It is impossible to mention the names of all the colleagues to whom I am indebted for their critical comments and constructive suggestions. All I can say is that had I not had the chance to read their works and discuss with them so many points, this book would never have been written. Nevertheless, I am extremely pleased to address special thanks to at least three of them, for their important contributions to my personal and scientific development. With his scientific work, valuable suggestions, and generous encouragements, John Bowlby has long been an inspiring model of scientific attitudes and clinical wisdom. I am also grateful to Walter B. Weimer for the epistemological and methodological rigor he has evoked in me each time we have met. Finally, I thank Michael J. Mahoney for the brotherly friendship with which he always turns our scientific discussions into something more special and unique.

PREFACE

This work belongs to a trend of research initiated over 10 years ago and directed toward the development of a scientific model of cognitive psychotherapy. Throughout many years of clinical practice and research, I have come to believe that a comprehensive model of human psychopathology is essential for the elaboration of reliable psychotherapeutic strategies. On the other hand, up to this moment psychology has traditionally addressed clinical disturbances primarily within a descriptive and dispositional framework whose main aim was to reduce the complexity and variability of emotional disorders by compressing them into a range of suitable terms and labels. Even though in the last decade some brilliant and promising cognitive approaches have made their appearance (Beck, 1976; Dobson, in press; Goldfried, 1982; Guidano & Liotti, 1983; Mahoney, 1980, in press; Meichenbaum, 1977; Reda & Mahoney, 1984), the psychotherapeutic field continues to be an ambiguous domain whose scientific ground remains questionable.

Accordingly, I am convinced of the growing need for cognitive psychologists to address more of their clinical research to the elaboration of a unitary, developmental, process-oriented model of psychopathology. Such a model would seek to assess the processes and conditions that give rise to specific individual knowledge organizations that when unbalanced, produce the patterns we commonly call clinical disturbances. In order to move in this direction, however, I found it necessary to make some basic choices, from both epistemological and methodological points of view.

Relevant to my epistemological premise are the limits inherent to an empiricist–associationist paradigm—a model that still bears so much influence on contemporary psychology. The shortcomings of this paradigm primarily reside in an overly simplistic conception of man and the world. If we assume that the order with which we are acquainted is given and belongs as such to reality, then the human mind becomes simply a passive receptor of this outside order and is determined by it more or less entirely (Bever, Fodor, & Garrrett, 1968; Hayek, 1952; Liotti & Reda, 1981; Mahoney, 1984; Weimer, 1977). This perspective, while presenting the indubitable qualities of simplicity and parsimony, also has the undeniable disadvantage of making all the more intractable the understanding of higher mental processes that is essential to the elaboration of any comprehensive model of psychopathology.

Over the last decade, primarily within the natural sciences, a totally different perspective has emerged that might instead be termed an "epistemology of complexity." According to this perspective, the ordering of reality is an inherent principle of the dynamics of life itself and therefore assumes growing forms of complexity as it proceeds along the evolutionary scale (Atlan, 1979, 1981; Gould, 1977, 1980; Jantsch, 1980; Jantsch & Waddington, 1976; Morin, 1977; Prigogine, 1980; Weimer, 1982b). In this context, *complexity* does not mean "complication," which is a limit to knowledge and understandability. This common meaning of the word is applicable only if we take for granted that simplicity— that is, to regard a living organism as a passive respondent to the environment—is the "normal" form of reality. On the contrary, to consider living organisms in terms of complexity means to emphasize from the very start their self-determination and self-organization, as well as the openness and plasticity of their evolutionary and developmental pathways. One hardly needs to point out that such an approach to human behavior is not a new theory or discipline, but rather a way of seeing things—a paradigm or reference frame in which already available observational and experimental data can be reconsidered in a more holistic and dynamic perspective.

From a methodological point of view, a stance toward human mental functioning in terms of complexity implies the assumption of a systems/process-oriented methodology—that is, an approach that not only takes into account the multiplicity of levels of analysis within a complex unit but also attempts to grasp the network of reciprocal intercorrelations underlying its wholeness (Lazslo, 1972, 1983; Lerner, Skinner, & Sorell, 1980; Levine, 1982; Sameroff, 1982). Such analysis is purely structural and explanatory in nature, rather than merely dispositional and descriptive like the ones commonly employed in associationistic–behavioristic inquiry (Weimer, 1979,

1984). From a methodological standpoint, the attainment of an explanatory level is a fundamental problem of contemporary psychology, as Weimer (1982b) has clearly stated:

> Mature sciences are explanatory rather than descriptive. Explanation consists in rendering intelligible how and why the phenomena within a domain exhibit the properties that, descriptively, they do possess. Science explains by conjecturing theories (either tacitly or in explicit, after-the-fact construction) that tell why things must be as they are observed to be. Psychologists, in contrast, have limited their accounts to dispositional analysis of the psychological domain. Dispositional analysis is at the best descriptive and cannot be considered explanatory. It is thus incumbent upon psychology to develop the sort of explanatory theory that mature sciences possess—theories that will derive surface-structure appearances lawfully from an abstract, deep-structural realm that is causally productive of those appearances. (pp. 336–337)

This book, therefore, represents an account of a search for a developmental and unitary model of human psychopathology carried out within the perspective of a systems/process-oriented approach to organized complexity.

Part I is briefly concerned with the basic epistemological and theoretical principles underlying the whole research. While Chapter 1 presents the important assumptions of an epistemology of complexity and the derivative methodological principles relevant to a systems approach, the following two chapters take into consideration the fundamental theoretical aspects that can be deduced from such epistemological underpinnings.

Chapter 2 introduces a perspective on knowledge processes useful in trying to explain the progressive development of higher levels of order and organized complexity usually exhibited by human mental functioning. Weimer's motor theory of the mind and Pribram's holographic model of information processing are the major interlocking themes around which the whole prospect revolves.

As a conclusion to Part I, Chapter 3 addresses the question of how a viewpoint based on complexity considers the self. Plainly, the approach to the self is very dissimilar from proposed self-concept theories whose basic attempt is to enlarge the empiricist–associationistic paradigm through the inclusion of centralized cognitive mediators of behavior (see Broughton & Reigel, 1977). The main difference consists in regarding the self not as a self-concept (i.e., like an entity connecting experience and behavior),

but as a concept of selfhood continuously remodeling and restructuring itself—that is, as a *process* accounting for the central feature
of human knowledge: its reflexive nature. Finally, since adequate
growth and integration of human knowledge is predicated on the
presence of others, Bowlby's attachment theory is presented as
the basic thread integrating the development and organization of
personal reality.

Part II is dedicated to developmental and organizational models
that can be elaborated on the basis of the previously outlined
theoretical framework.

Chapter 4 proposes a unitary model of selfhood development
that relies on a multilevel method of analysis. This model not only
attempts to take into consideration the interdependence between
cognitive growth and emotional differentiation but also describes
various family and environmental conditions that act on this
cognitive–emotional interdependence. In fact, clinical psychologists
are now more and more inclined to recognize the need to construct
integrative models in order to explain the interdependence between
affect and cognition (cf. Greenberg & Safran, 1984). In this perspective, and in accordance with other supporters of a systems
approach methodology (Sameroff, 1982), I believe that concepts
such as "scripts" (Abelson, 1981; Schank & Abelson, 1977) in general,
and "nuclear scripts" (Tomkins, 1978) in particular, represent
promising tools of integration that may serve to account for the
interaction between feeling and thinking throughout the developmental process. Clinical vignettes introduced in Chapter 4 and
continuing throughout the rest of the book are not intended to
give the reader detailed clinical or diagnostic descriptions, but
rather are meant to exemplify the developmental aspects of this
model through instances of real life.

To conclude Part II, Chapter 5 outlines the general structural
organization of knowledge processes that acquires increasing stability by the end of the maturational stages. The basic idea, and
the foundation for the subsequent chapters, is the concept of "personal cognitive organization," that is, specific arrangement of personal meaning processes by which each individual is provided
with a sense of oneness and historical continuity in the course of
his/her lifespan. The most relevant difference between this and
other personality models is embodied in the fact that basic regulative
mechanisms are no longer connected to motivational aspects

(whether meant as drives or hedonistic determinism) but to *cognitive* aspects. Thus the essential mechanism of self-regulation is identified by the tendency to maintain the systemic coherence of one's personal meaning processes. The resulting image of the human being is no longer that of a hedonistic animal whose behavior is regulated step-by-step by rewards and punishments, but rather that of an epistemologic animal whose adaptive adequacy coincides with the effectiveness of his/her understanding of self and reality.

Lastly, Part III is entirely devoted to the exposition of a developmental, process-oriented model of psychopathology consistent with the theoretical and methodologic principles expressed in the preceding parts.

Chapter 6 examines the general patterns and processes that, during the maturational stages, contribute to the development of personal cognitive organizations marked by a high degree of internal incongruities and therefore particularly subject to the specific disequilibriums known as clinical disorders. Chapters 7, 8, 9, and 10 analyze in greater detail the four types of personal cognitive organization most frequently found in psychotherapeutic practice— depressive, phobic, eating disorders, and obsessive organizations. Developmental and organizational aspects of each of these are considered with special emphasis on the fact that the onset of a cognitive dysfunction is always related to exceedingly rigid and stereotyped mechanisms of maintenance of one's systemic coherence.

Chapter 11 concludes Part III with an outline of some general principles of lifespan developmental psychopathology. In particular, the growing sense of irreversibility in one's *temporal becoming*, which is progressively observed during the course of an individual lifespan, is believed to be at the origin of deep, challenging transformations in one's personal reality. Additionally, the effect of such transformations may be to facilitate the onset of clear-cut clinical syndromes in personal cognitive organizations that may lie on a narrow-margin equilibrium.

As a conclusion to the book, I have outlined some fundamental principles of psychotherapeutic strategy that can be deduced on the basis of this model of psychopathology.

V. F. G.

CONTENTS

Any attempt to conceive persons completely as a kind of thing in the world persisting through time will come up against this obstacle. The self that appears to the subject seems to disappear under external analysis.—Nagel (1979)

PART ONE

THEORETICAL PRINCIPLES

CHAPTER ONE

INTRODUCTORY NOTES ON SELF-ORGANIZED COMPLEXITY AND A SYSTEMS APPROACH

. . . the living being from the bacterium to homo sapiens, obeys a particular logic according to which the individual, though ephemeral, singular, and marginal, considers itself the center of the world. All others are excluded from the individual's ontological site, including homozygous twins, congeners, fellowmen. According to a law of exclusion that brings to mind Pauli's principle, this egocentricity, which excludes from itself all other beings, this computation and ethos *for the self* furnishes the logical, organizational, and existential definition of the concept of *subject.*—Morin (1981)

In the last decade, an evolutionary, holistic, and process-oriented perspective to living systems has directed special attention to such concepts as hierarchical organization, temporal becoming, and dynamic equilibrium. This focus has led to the conceptualization of the human knowing system as a self-referent, organized complexity whose distinctive hallmark is its self-organizing ability (Atlan, 1981; Jantsch, 1980; Jantsch & Waddington, 1976; Laszlo, 1972, 1983; Nicolis & Prigogine, 1977; Prigogine, 1980; Varela, 1979; Weimer, 1982a, 1983).

The essential feature of this perspective considers the self-organizing ability of a human knowing system as a basic evolutionary constraint that, through the maturational ascension of higher cognitive abilities, progressively structures a full sense of self-identity with inherent feelings of uniqueness and historical continuity. The availability of this stable and structured self-identity permits continuous and coherent self-perception and self-evaluation in the face of temporal becoming and mutable reality. For this reason, the maintenance of one's perceived identity becomes as important as life itself; without it the individual would be incapable of proper functioning and would lose, at the same time, the very sense of reality.

A self-organized knowing system is *autonomous* for at least two fundamental reasons. First, one's perceived self-identity is not simply received from an external reality already "objectively" ordered, but is *actively* constructed by the knowing subject who produces his/her own identity by ordering ongoing experience according to available information-processing capabilities. Thus, the world is interpreted and dealt with differently not only in relation to one's distinct personality organization, but also in reference to the particular developmental stage in which an individual is currently functioning.

Secondly, all the possible pressures for change that emerge as a consequence of the ongoing assimilation of experience are subordinate to the maintenance of one's identity—the fundamental self-organizing invariant. Though one experiences changes in his/her "parts" throughout the lifespan, the individual *as a whole* maintains his/her perceived identity over time. Maintenance takes place through the individual's "autopoietic activity"—a concept derived from *autopoiesis*, a Greek word meaning self-production or self-renewal (Varela, 1979; Zeleny, 1981). That is, through an ongoing, generative process of self-renewal, perturbations arising from exchanges with the world are transformed into more complex and integrated levels of self-identity and self-consciousness.

The notion of autonomous computation arising from this context seems particularly important. If *autonomy* is defined in terms of "systemic self-reference," it can be easily distinguished from the usual metaphysical definitions in terms of "freedom," "indeterminacy," or "irrationality." Thus, in order to maintain or renew itself, a self-organized complexity needs nothing else but reference to itself.

The consequent differentiation between *autonomy* ("self-law") and *allonomy* ("external law") could hold special relevance for a better understanding of current debates between different trends in cognitive psychology. An autonomous system such as the human mind, unlike an input–output device, is a self-referent individual unit of perception and action that maintains internally generated reference levels (Varela, 1976a). Therefore, above all it refers to a function coming from itself and is not aimed at the production of any specific output. Instead, it is concerned with its own self-maintenance and self-renewal.

In contrast, an allonomous input–output processing system (e.g., a computer) relies on a function coming from the outside—

a program—in order to produce some specific output. A computer, therefore, besides having a very limited ability to reconstruct and renew itself, has an allonomous computation because it produces experience whose meaningfulness is defined by external parameters and consequently is subordinate to the production of something different from itself. This is why, according to Pask (1981), there should be no need to ask ourselves *why* there are self-referent, autopoietic systems—they *are* the units of reality. The cogent question is whether there are any allopoietic systems except those engendered and engineered by the static artifice of a "program" (p. 301).

On the other hand, viewing a human knowing system as a self-organized complexity is not at all a sort of new theory or discipline, but rather a *paradigm*—that is, a conceptual framework to understand the recursive intercorrelation that connects each part of the system to the others. Indeed, the Latin word *complexus* originally meant "different elements interlaced together to form a single fabric." Therefore, the paradigm of complexity, by defining the wholeness of a system in terms of self-organization, recursiveness, dynamic equilibrium, and so on, aims essentially at transforming the study of holism and wholeness into a legitimate field of inquiry for the natural sciences. Such an approach also represents a clear demarcation from the metaphysical notions frequently employed in its study thus far.

Finally, once a complexity perspective is adopted, a systems/process-oriented approach consequently becomes a preferential methodology of inquiry in order to grasp the network of reciprocal correlations underlying wholeness. Therefore, in the sections that follow, I shall briefly explain the main theoretical and methodological aspects to which I have tried to adhere during the course of this whole exposition.

EVOLUTIONARY EPISTEMOLOGY

In recent years, epistemology (the study of knowledge processes and knowing systems) has progressively become a discipline unto itself, consistent with the characteristics of the scientific method. However, it does not seem as yet to have influenced psychologists as much as one might have expected. The reason for this is probably that in keeping with the prevailing empiricist–behavioristic perspective, which reduces the study of psychology to the description of interactions between organism and environment, many psychologists are still convinced that questions regarding the origin and nature of knowledge belong solely to such fields as philosophy and metaphysics.

In contrast, Weimer (1982b), has suggested that epistemology, having supplied a true falsifiable approach for understanding the nature of our knowledge as well as the manner of its acquisition, should be considered with full right one of the psychological sciences. In particular the branch called evolutionary epistemology seems to hold special relevance for cognitive psychology. The application of an evolutionary perspective to the growth of knowledge seems to reveal that knowledge itself—being the emerging result of biological and adaptive processes—has evolved along with other aspects of life (Campbell, 1974; Lorenz, 1973; Piaget, 1971; Popper, 1972; Popper & Eccles, 1977).

In other words, within an adaptive perspective, "knowledge" becomes a biological as well as psychological process and is defined once and for all as a specific field of natural science. I also am in agreement with Weimer (1982b) in asserting that evolutionary epistemology should form the basis for any consistent cognitive psychology methodology. This would not only help resolve some of the debated issues concerning the relationship between knowledge and reality, but would also tend to elucidate the higher, self-organized role that knowledge progressively assumes as a result of an increase in evolutionary complexity. Additionally, this would serve to point the way to further inquiry. Let us consider for a moment the general characteristics of these aspects.

The notion that knowledge structures are evolutionary patterns of information gathering and processing, progressively scaffolded in response to challenging environmental pressures, implies that the organism's *activity* is the key feature of its interaction with the world (Popper, 1975).

> All organisms are problem solvers. They are constantly engaged, day and night, in solving many problems. Of course, they are unconscious problem solvers. . . . All these problems have a direction: they are all attempts to anticipate the future. . . . Thus, from a very early stage, problem solving and anticipation or theory construction about the environment play a central part in the behavior of organisms. They remain central throughout the whole range of higher organisms;

especially, of course, of higher animals, including man. (Popper, 1982, pp. 45–46)

Since ordering and decoding are the essential devices for effective survival, knowledge evolution appears as an unfolding process, characterized by the progressive scaffolding of even more complex environment-modeled templates capable of ordering and decoding ongoing experience. In short, organisms are "theories of their environment", as Weimer (1975) cogently put it.

All this, of course, implies a dramatic change in our traditional viewpoint of the relationship between knowledge and reality. Knowledge can no longer be regarded as an approximation to truth—that is, as a step forward in grasping an ultimate and certain reality—since knowledge simply expresses a specific relationship between knower and known (Sameroff, 1982).

> Hence, this world of ours, no matter how we structure it, no matter how well we manage to keep it stable with permanent objects and recurrent interactions, is by definition a world codependent with our experience, and not the ontological reality of which philosophers and scientists alike have dreamed. (Varela, 1979, p. 275)

Therefore, knowledge, being a theory of the environment to which the organism has adapted, always reflects the specific self-referent constraints through which the organism scaffolds its own reality. As Aaronson (1972) points out, we structure the world in terms of our body image; we are three-dimensional organisms characterized by front–back, right–left, and top–bottom, and we structure space in terms of height, width, and depth. Moreover, having a sense of self that is perceived as individuality and uniqueness, we are similarly led to consider entirely natural the ordering of reality within a set of circumscribed entities to which we attribute such individuality. These become all the more meaningful to us when we attribute to them the same kind of phenomena that we experience directly, that is, drives and intentions. In other words, the tendency to scaffold ongoing experience in an anthropomorphic form is apparently just as natural to us as it is to attribute spatial qualities to the surrounding world.

In an evolutionary epistemology perspective, knowledge and mindlike behaviors appear to be an immanent quality of every living system, capable of assuming different levels of organized complexity according to their respective evolutionary levels. As Pribram (1980a) clearly argues:

> Mind so defined, is an emergent property of information processing by the brain much as wetness is an emergent property of the appropriate organization of hydrogen and oxygen into water, and gravity is an emergent property of the organization of matter into interacting masses. (p. 60)

If mind appears to be distributed along a continuum ranging from early rudimentary exploratory behaviors to human self-consciousness, then evolution emerges as an essential *regulation strategy* aimed at achieving stability in an ever-changing environment through attainment of more complex levels of autonomous, self-referent functioning. In other words, organized complexity and self-organization seem to have been interwoven ever since their first appearance and, consequently, the specific patterns and processes underlying the emergence of our perceived identity can be confidently regarded as stemming from the evolutionary and systemic constraints underlying our mental processing.

> Selfhood is a necessary consequence of structurally complex systems that satisfy certain constraints. That we know selves as embodied by the highest primates is, in effect, due to local factors in this region of universe; selves could be embodied quite differently. (Weimer, 1982b, p. 352)

HIERARCHICAL ORGANIZATION AND COALITIONAL CONTROL

The evolution of autonomous, self-organizing units is made possible by the parallel structuring of hierarchical systems whose level of organization varies according to the corresponding level of organized complexity achieved by the system (cf. Pattee, 1973). An organization consists of a multilevel ensemble of reciprocally interacting subsystems differentiated on the basis of their structure and function, and hierarchically arranged to ensure the system a level of coordination and integration necessary for the maintenance of its individuality. The exclusive preeminence acquired by hierarchical organizations in the course of evolution of living systems can be readily explained with the consideration that such organizations are able to provide a system with greater plasticity and adaptive adequacy toward a dynamic, continuously changing environment.

> Systems that are based on hierarchies are much more stable, because failure in organization will not destroy the whole system but only decompose it to the next stable subsystem level. As a consequence, instead of starting all over again, the process of complexification can start from the stable subsystem level and reconstitute the loss in a much shorter period of time. (Sameroff, 1982, p. 97)

Furthermore, what characterizes the degree of flexibility and plasticity of a system is the way control is distributed within its hierarchical organization. The more a system exhibits decentralized control instead of a single "executive" center, the more likely it is that continuous shiftings in the relations among subsystems will occur, allowing them to modify their reciprocal cooperation in a variety of ways depending on the context or sphere of action involved. No wonder, then, that the emergence of higher, self-organized units accompanied by even more sophisticated patterns of decentralization make the human knowing system one of the most admirable and complex examples of coalitional control of a hierarchical organization (Shaw & McIntyre, 1974).

> The person (CNS) as a whole seems to be a coalition of (perhaps) hierarchical structures, somehow allied together but with no single locus in ultimate control, even when observable behavior appears to be exclusively occupied with one task, or when conscious awareness says "I am in charge." There is cooperation and mutual coordination, a context of interacting constraint, but no single control center. Decentralization of control is one of the definitive properties of coalitions. A second is the lack of a determinantly specifiable boundary between the coordinated systems. Clearly perception is not memory or locomotion, but one cannot sharply separate any of the three. Thus the boundaries of a coalition both as a whole and within itself are intrinsically "fuzzy." A third crucial property is that coalitional structures are superadditive. As the Gestalt phrase goes, the whole is more than the additive sum of its parts. What the coalition can "do" is vastly greater than any of its components, even when the latter are individually summed up. (Weimer, 1983, p. 15)

What methodological framework can be adopted from a perspective where mind is seen as a multilevel coalition of quite independent, though interlocked, self-referent structures and processes? In order to address the productivity, multilinearity, and multidirectionality of human knowing processes, it has been suggested that an adequate systems approach methodology will have to be based upon a *multiple level of analysis* (Lerner *et al.*, 1980; Levine, 1982; Sameroff, 1982). In other words, the researcher will have to be able to operate, at any time, simultaneously on different levels of analysis, both in selecting significant observational data and in testing hypotheses arising from attempts to find adequate explanations for such data.

DYNAMIC EQUILIBRIUM AND DIALECTICAL GROWTH

A self-organized unit may be viewed as a growing system whose lifespan development is regulated by the principle of orthogenetic progression; meaning that the system proceeds toward more integrated levels of structural order and complexity (Werner, 1948, 1957).

This conception of living systems, in spite of being supported by experience and common sense, typically has been met with skepticism by the scientific community. This fact can be largely attributed to the pervasive influence of the thermodynamic principles of classical physics that hold just the opposite view—that is, that a physical system left to itself, in time faces growing disorder and final disintegration. As a consequence of this adherence to the classic physics paradigm (which is more or less tacitly endorsed by most traditional psychological trends), the consideration of directionality and generative progression in development has been excluded. By and large, development has characteristically been depicted as a sort of passive and cumulative process regulated at any moment by contingency relationships established with the environment.

In the last 15 years, the development of irreversible thermodynamics of self-organizing units has provided support for an alternative conception of physical and biological systems (Brent, 1978b; Nicolis & Prigogine, 1977; Prigogine, 1976, 1978, 1980). According to this view, the key property underlying autonomy of any form of self-organization resides in a system's ability to turn into self-referent order the randomness of perturbations coming either from the environment or from internal oscillations ("order-from-noise" principle; Atlan, 1981).

The temporal evolution of a human knowing system also appears to possess a generative, nonlinear directionality marked by the discontinuous emerging of more complex and integrated levels of self-identity and self-consciousness. The principle underlying this dynamic equilibrium has been termed "order through fluctuations," for higher order patterns emerge through the assimilation of disequilibriums (fluctuations) arising from interaction with the environment. Each time a fluctuation becomes amplified to such an extent that it oversteps the existing range of stability, the emerging disequilibrium drives the system in the direction of restructuring its self-referent ordering processes.

The crucial feature of a self-stabilizing system is found not so much in the preservation of homeostatic, circular equilibrium, but rather in the maintenance of the *coherence* of one's ordering processes by means of continuous equilibrium restructurings. I agree with Dell (1982) who contends that an adequate systems approach methodology aimed at understanding the temporal stability of a self-organizing unit should seek to replace the concept of homeostasis with one of maintenance of systemic coherence.

Finally, it is important to point out that the notion of order through fluctuations clearly implies the constant presence of a rhythmic and essential tension among simultaneous but opponent processes of maintenance and change. Indeed, "opponent process regulation" seems to be a distinctive hallmark of human knowing systems and can be regarded as a logical consequence of their coalitional control (Weimer, 1983). Within a multilevel ensemble of differentiated but interconnected processes, decentralization of control can more conveniently take place if the opponent ordering processes come to regulate each other through complementary relationships. Though distinct, these relationships mutually specify and control one another. Oscillations and contradictions that constantly emerge from this network of opponent–complementary relationships lead the system to restructure its equilibrium in order to maintain its internal coherence. Since any self-organizing system evolves toward greater complexity and structural order by assimilating its own incongruities and contradictions, growth and development are inherently dialectical (Lerner & Busch-Rossnagel, 1981; Lerner *et al.*, 1980; Riegel, 1976, 1979; Sameroff, 1982).

As a result, an adequate systems approach strategy to study the essential tension between opponent processes requires that the investigator be able to view the binary oppositions exhibited by an organized complexity as irreducible components of the system. Thus, instead of looking at each of the opponent polarities in search of the true one, the investigator, through the reconstruction of *patterns* of recursive circularity among polarities, can formulate a hypothesis about the kind of internal coherence exhibited by the system (Pattee, 1982; Varela, 1976b, 1984).

TEMPORAL BECOMING AND THE HISTORICAL DIMENSION

Becoming is a passage from the future to the past. It is located at the present. — Watanabe (1972)

The orthogenetic progression of a self-organizing system unfolds embracing an irreversible temporal direction. According to Prigogine (1973), "irreversibility" should be understood as a symmetry-breaking process—that is, a break of the symmetry between past and future. With irreversibility we enter the domain of processes and the world becomes historic, resting on a temporal order— that is, the time direction from the past into the future. We experience this order as the "objective" temporal dimension—something belonging to reality rather than just to our subjective sense.

Perception of an irreversible directedness of time is essential in the structuring of human experience. This perception forms the foundation of our sense of causality and its characteristic directionality, which always has the cause preceding the consequence, never vice versa. The evolutionary meaning of such temporal ordering can be readily grasped when we consider that a sense of direction, either from past to present or present to future, is a fundamental requisite for developing effective goal-seeking behavior. As Atlan (1979) pointed out, the principle of irreversibility of time corresponds to the principle of primacy of action in adaptive processes.

Even in structuring a relationship with time, the progressive autonomy of a self-organized complexity from its environment is matched by the establishment of an autonomous inner world. In fact, the ontogeny of a self-organizing unit begins with the system's ability to extract meaningful information from the perceived temporal flux, and to scaffold this information into its individual temporal order. In other words, throughout the developmental lifespan, time directedness is projected into cognitive processes. This brings forth an internal structural transformation of time by which each human knowing system has its own inner "subjective" time, flowing parallel and interwoven with the perceived "objective" temporal order.

Moreover, by considering the entire lifespan development of a human knowing system, changes can be identified in its subjective experience of time similar to Prigogine's symmetry-breaking processes—that is, progressive irreversible differentiations between one's sense of past and future. Indeed, each lifespan starts with virtual total temporal symmetry—an exclusive sense of present in infancy and childhood stemming from an immediate experiencing of oneself and reality. Only after adolescence does breaking give way to a growing distinction between past and future. Through the discontinuous emergence of further symmetry-breaking processes, individual temporal becoming unfolds, leading to a progressive restructuring of the subjective experience of past and future. Needless to say, any transformation in one's experiencing of existential time produces a new space–time dimension and consequently initiates considerable changes in one's sense of self and the world. These changes have great influence on the oscillations and the course of the subsequent lifespan. Temporal evolution is open not only in regard to its products, but also in relation to the rules of the game it develops (Jantsch, 1980).

If we consider a human being as not only a knowing system, but also as a *historical* knowing system, the immediate methodological consequence is that a systems approach should employ a *lifespan developmental perspective*. This is because the systemic coherence of any self-organizing unit can be understood only by taking into consideration the system's starting boundary conditions and its subsequent developmental pathway.

Having related the essentials of a systems/process-oriented approach, the next two chapters shall complete our account of the theoretical perspective that occupies Part I of this book. The first of these chapters is an analysis of patterns and processes that characterize human knowledge, whereas the second focuses on epistemological principles and psychological processes underlying the development and maintenance of the self—that is, *who* has that knowledge.

CHAPTER TWO

A MOTOR–EVOLUTIONARY PERSPECTIVE ON HUMAN KNOWLEDGE

Once one abandons simpleminded perspectives such as behaviorism or information theory, it becomes obvious that the human higher mental processes are among the most complex and intractable problems known to man. Even the simplest behaviors are the result of enormously complex and abstract causal processes that result, in last analysis, from the central nervous system's ability to structure and restructure its own activity. —Weimer (1974)

MOTOR THEORIES OF THE MIND

Rather than being a mere reflection of a reality given to us by the external world, the familiar order and regularity of our phenomenal experience—including the richness of our sensory experiences— are the product of the active, self-referent capabilities of the human mind. Therefore, the sensory order can best be understood as a self-organized, classifying-decoding mechanism that orders and stabilizes the ongoing inflow through the detection of the highly abstract patterns of its own activity. These patterns of regularity are termed sensory qualities. In Pribram's words (1982b): "Brain, by organizing the input from the physical world, as obtained through the senses, constructs mental properties" (p. 29).

Hayek (1978), with his notion of the "primacy of the abstract," has emphasized that the richness of the sensory world we experience is not the starting point from which the mind derives abstractions. Conversely, it is the product of a great range of abstractions that the mind must possess in order to be capable of experiencing that richness of detail. What has been taken for granted in explaining the functioning of the mind—that the concrete seems primary while the abstract appears to be derived from it—appears to be an error of our subjective experience reflecting the complex ordering constraints that the human mind has acquired in the course of its evolutionary history (Hayek, 1952).[1]

> Sense experience therefore presupposes the existence of a sort of accumulated "knowledge," of an acquired order of the sensory impulses based on their past co-occurrence; and this knowledge, although based on (pre-sensory) experience, can never be contradicted by sense experiences and will determine the forms of such experiences which are possible. (Hayek, 1952, p. 167)

In an evolutionary epistemology perspective, the mind appears to be an active, constructive system, capable of producing not only its output but also, to a large extent, the input it receives—including the basic sensations underlying the construction of itself. That is why, in recent years, there has been a growing need to shift the conceptualization of the mind toward "motor theories" (Weimer, 1977) and to drop conventional empiricist sensory theories that depict the mind as a mere collector of sensations, which implies the rather simplistic assumption that the order and method with which we are acquainted actually belong to reality.

From a motor theory perspective, information processing (input) and behavior (output) are no longer considered functionally distinct, for sensory functions are construed as mediated by the same neural pathways as motor functions.[2] For example, the structures underlying the production of speech are presumed to underlie its comprehension (Halwes & Wire, 1974). Accordingly, processes underlying perception are believed to be identical to those underlying imagination, just as thought processes are viewed as inseparable from motor activity. Hence we do not first think and then act, since cognitive processes are themselves actions. Piaget (1970) stated many years ago that to know an object means to accommodate and assimilate it into one's ongoing level of expectations, which, in the final analysis, essentially means to act upon it.

In a motor theory perspective, mental functioning is no longer characterized by the making and breaking of associative ties derived from the passive acquisition of chronological (i.e., classical conditioning) or consequential (i.e., operant conditioning) contingency relationships. In contrast, it is an ongoing matching process through which a neural model of the environment is continuously updated by comparison with the incoming sensory inflow (Pribram, 1971). Modeling the external reality—as well as its own internal activity—is the fundamental self-referent function of the nervous system. This modeling process determines the very form that experience can assume because any stimulus whose occurrence could not be matched against a neural model for detecting regularities could never be perceived by our senses.

Furthermore, in order to scaffold any stimulus into a specific sensation, the nervous system must match and mismatch it to an internalized model of that sensation. Thus, the classifying–decoding activity involved in any aspect of our mental processing is carried out by contrast enhancement. As Mahoney (1982) has pointed out, the most striking aspect of the human quest for meaning consists, essentially, in seeking order through contrast, an instance, we may assume, of an oscillatory and complementary relationship between opponent ordering processes. Therefore, the abstract rules for detecting regularities and invariances reflect the self-referent, classificatory activity of the nervous system, rather than intrinsic properties of the real world. Furthermore, these rules are the result of neural modeling that represents a match-to-pattern procedure carried out by opponent processes regulation (Weimer, 1983).

The emergence of verbal conscious thought increased both the complexity and the flexibility of neural classificatory activity. This development allowed a system to monitor and act upon its immediate apprehension of reality, either through performing a closer analysis of some specific aspect or by effecting a particular modification deemed necessary. As Weimer (1982a) stated: "The nervous system as a hierarchically organized instrument of classification leads to the conception of conscious thought as an evolutionarily programmed fail-safe device for reclassification" (p. 269). In other words, in moving toward ever higher levels of organized complexity, the autonomy of an evolving self-referent unit from its environment becomes increasingly related to a disengagement from the *immediacy* of its experience of the environment.

Thus in a motor–evolutionary perspective, tacit and explicit aspects of knowing are the expression of two closely interconnected levels of cognitive processes. Tacit–abstract processes provide the apperceptive scaffolding through which conscious, selective attention is constrained, allowing the insertion and manipulation of deep ordering rules into explicit procedures of thought representations—for example, theories, beliefs, problem-solving strategies, and so on. The most remarkable consequence of this conception of mind regards the central role played by unconscious processes (Franks, 1974; Polanyi, 1966; Reber & Lewis, 1977; Shevrin & Dickman, 1980; Turvey, 1974; Weimer, 1973, 1974, 1977). From this viewpoint, tacit processes are seen as the higher hierarchical level. Far from being a "sub-conscious" level, they are actually a "superconscious" one, because they govern conscious processes without appearing in them. In Hayek's (1978) terms, products of conscious rationality are the result of human actions, but not of human design.

Since tacit and explicit aspects of knowing will be a central theme throughout the rest of this exposition, let us develop the subject in a more detailed manner.

TACIT AND EXPLICIT LEVELS OF KNOWING

Data emerging from experimental psychology in the last decades have suggested the existence of preconscious, anticipatory cognitive structures that direct the focus of conscious selective attention. Concepts like Bartlett's "schemata" (1932) or the "mental sets" so widely used by information-processing approaches (see Miller, Galanter, & Pribram, 1960) are but a few examples. However, only in recent years, with the availability of a motor–evolutionary approach to knowledge processes (Hayek, 1952, 1978; Weimer, 1977, 1982a), new perspectives in neurophysiology and neuropsychology (Pribram, 1971, 1977), and epistemological approaches reproposing the problem of knowing as recognizing (Kuhn, 1970; Lakatos, 1974; Polanyi, 1966; Weimer, 1973), have we been allowed to collect within a unitary framework data and hypotheses concerning conscious and unconscious processes.

In order to further clarify the distinction between tacit and explicit aspects of knowing, the role of these processes will be reviewed within the contexts of: (1) an evolutionary perspective; (2) recent neuropsychological models of information processing; and (3) individual lifespan development.

The Evolutionary Perspective

From an evolutionary viewpoint, the problem of distinguishing two levels of knowing processes only appears in the human species and may be best exemplified by the emergence of language and the specialization of the cerebral hemispheres.

Although the evolutionary significance of the differentiation between cerebral hemispheres has yet to be fully appreciated, and the mechanisms that led to its emergence are still obscure, it is clear that hemispheric specialization is unique to human beings. Primates do not show any apparent sign of differentiation in their hemispheres, which appear symmetric both structurally and functionally. It has been suggested that, until this level of evolution, the development of a bilaterally symmetric brain has been a sort of evolutionary fail-safe device for maximizing adaptation (Passingham, 1982; Springer & Deutsch, 1981). In effect, a double mirror structure is still capable of maintaining an integrated level of functioning, even if a portion of it is seriously damaged. For example, with one hemisphere totally removed, monkeys are still able to learn relatively complicated tasks with apparently normal facility (Nakamura & Gazzaniga, 1978).

The break in symmetry occurs in human evolution in response to unique demands and specific pressures imposed by the emergence of the unprecedented evolutionary challenge represented by language. Indeed, language afforded such autonomy from the environment as to vastly compensate for the loss of advantages related to a symmetric brain. On the one hand, it becomes possible to *reify* the ongoing immediate apprehension of reality, bordering and structuring it in entities that, as concepts, have stability and consistency, and can therefore be manipulated, figuratively speaking, on the same level as real objects (Bronowski & Bellugi, 1970; Popper & Eccles, 1977). On the other hand, the internalization of language, by yielding increasingly accurate and defined inner representation, gave way to sophisticated mental mapping abilities capable of modifying and adapting the immediate apprehension of reality to current plans of action. With this ability to reach beyond the perceptual field, human beings attained an unprecedented level of disengagement from the immediacy of experience and acquired new possibilities to explore and control the environment, as well as an ever increasing level of comprehension of themselves and the world.

Thus, the left hemisphere specialization for language has led to a consequent reorganization in which the assignment of different roles and functions to the two hemispheres reflects a basic separation of human higher mental processes (Davidson, 1980; Gazzaniga & LeDoux, 1978; Popper & Eccles, 1977; Sperry, 1982; Teuber, 1974). While the left hemisphere is specialized for sequential and analytic processes, the right hemisphere is more concerned with holistic and synthetic space–time relationships—that is, with the processing of unconscious, tacit information. As the final stage of the specialization process, the two hemispheres have reached a level of integrated functional unity by the structuring of a dynamic, complementary relationship. It is quite likely that, from the start, the functional complementarity of a left hemisphere specialized in analytical and logical tasks, and a right hemisphere specialized in holistic and emotional tasks, has considerably increased chances of adaptive adequacy.

With the advent of hemisphere specialization came the establishment of decentralized control whereby the moment-to-moment dominance of the entire system continuously oscillates between these two knowing dimensions. Within such an oscillative equilibrium, the conscious processing of this complementary specialization was assumed by emerging higher linguistic functions. This allowed for plans of action formulated in words to be adequately evaluated and efficiently executed under the conscious focus of the hemisphere specialized for language (Passingham, 1982).

In other words, it is as if a sort of "choice of the species" occurred, in which conscious executive control over environmental exploration was assigned to emerging logical–conceptual capabilities and the new possibilities that they offered. On the other hand, since the forms of preverbal knowledge appeared much earlier in the course of evolution, they are presumed to be more deeply rooted in the phylogenetic structure. As a result, one may logically posit that such tacit-forms of knowledge continued to function by providing a global, apprehensional frame whereby conscious control became focused upon extremely specialized, but for this very reason inevitably partial, higher cortical processes.

Holographic and Analytic Processing

For a number of years, Pribram (1971) has been calling attention to the fact that the nervous system employs two different forms of neural events for processing and transmitting information: continuous and discrete. Continuous events consist of the rhythmic modification of graded slow-potential waves coming from the junctional microstructure of neuronal aggregates, while discrete activities are the unitary, intermittent, intraneuronal discharges of all-or-none impulses.

Continuous events are believed to be phylogenetically older and consist of a spatial, "overall" codification of spontaneous neural activity. This is believed to be accomplished through the monitoring of the differences in the distribution of impulse patterns (interference wave patterns) existing in the brain at a given time. Discrete events appear in more and more differentiated ways as neural complexity increases and involve a temporal codification of sets of distinct neuronal firings patterned into a sequential rate of all-or-none spike potentials. Because the graded slow-potential activities are mechanisms for classifying and decoding the continuous interactions among interference wave patterns, they essentially follow an analogical logic (i.e., comparison and contrast). Intraneuronal discharges, on the other hand, are intermittent and based solely on a binary code (all-or-none), and therefore follow a digital or analytical logic. Furthermore, these two neural events are entirely interconnected, for the graded slow-potential activity represents the fundamental mechanism capable of "reading" the sequential rates of spike potentials occurring in any part of the brain.

Pribram not only has provided researchers with a descriptive neurophysiological framework delineating how differences in the electrical activity of the brain can support the presence of analogical and analytical codes as well as their reciprocal intercorrelation, but also has proposed a *holographic* model to explain the nature of graded slow potentials and of the interference wave patterns that derive from them (Pribram, 1971, 1977, 1980a, 1980b, 1982a, 1982b, 1986).

"Holography" refers to several methods developed within the field of optical information processing for producing and storing distributed information and reproducing it in a three-dimensional way (Gabor, 1972). There are a number of parallels between the properties of holograms and the brain's capacity for storing and retrieving information. Besides the readiness with which images can be reconstructed three-dimensionally from the information stored in the photographic plate, one of the most striking characteristics of holographic storage is its distributed information state—meaning that the whole of the image is reproduced within each of its parts. This property seems to make holograms, like the brain, highly resistant to damage. Further, this characteristic allows for a huge memory capacity (some hundred million bits of retrievable information in a cubic centimeter of holographic memory) and consequently increases quite dramatically the system's computational power.

A holographic model of the brain hypothesizes a number of key concepts. These concepts and their most important consequences can be outlined as follows.

1. Similar to optical holograms, the interference wave patterns derived from the graded slow-potential activity (distributed information) may generate a whole set of three-dimensional representations when connected with the appropriate "reference beam."

As Weimer (1982b) emphasized, a holographic model and its characteristic distributed information processing not only can explain the enormous amounts of holistic information contained at a deep tacit level, but can also account for the decentralization of control in such information. This would serve to explain the flexibility and generativity exhibited by many aspects of mental functioning. Indeed, from such an ensemble of holographic "images" or "schemata," an indefinitely extended domain of verbal and visual surface representations can be generated, depending on the quality of moment-to-moment experience. Considering these characteristics, it is clear how in the evolution of self-organized complexity, holographic storage may have become the most economic, sophisticated, and evolutionarily adaptive method for storing and retrieving information.

2. Another characteristic quality of information processing by holography is that once an image is reconstructed, it leaps out into a space away from the storage medium. This is analogous to two well-balanced stereo speakers whose sound seems to project from a point midway between them. The holographic "stereo effect," besides explaining the powerfulness and vividness of mental images, is also at present the most plausible explanation of the way consciousness of the self is typically experienced. For each one of us, our holistic felt identity stands out in a sort of kinesthetic point of reference, regulating and coordinating our conscious procedures of thought representations. As Pribram (1980a) pointed out:

> The holographic model (mathematical and optical) helps to explain
> how a brain process can give rise to an image which is experienced
> as remote from the representational mechanism and even the receptor
> surface which is involved in the construction of the image. The contents

of consciousness (what we are aware of) are thus experienced apart from the brain apparatus (holographic and control) that organizes those contents from its inputs. Mind and brain are separate except in this special relation to each other. (p. 59)

3. Increasing convergent evidence supports the hypothesis that the brain encodes sensory input in a holographic fashion. Over the past decade, a number of studies have shown that mathematical descriptions of sensory processes fit those described by holography (see Pribram, 1980b, for references). Therefore, it is the continuous modulation of interference wave patterns that gives rise to the tacit apperceptive scaffolding of ongoing experience that extends beyond the individual capability of paying attention.

In other words, the holographic hypothesis provides a neurophysiological model that embodies Hayek's primacy of the abstract and the richness of the sensory world deriving from it, and at the same time accounts for the implicit nature of experience. Dennett (1978) cogently stated that one perceives more than one experiences, experiences more than one attends to, and experiences more at any one time than one wants to say at that time.

As a result of the interconnections between holographic (tacit) and analytic (explicit) processing, the most salient aspects of the perceived global apprehension can be repeatedly placed in the focal conscious attention and transformed into explicit objects of thought—expectations, beliefs, problem-solving procedures, and so on. As Pribram (1977) explained, "The intrinsic properties, the implicate organization, is holographic. As extrinsic properties become realized, they make the implicate organization become more explicit" (p. 98).

Having seen that hemispheric specialization offers an evolutionary basis for the differentiation of tacit and explicit levels of knowing, and that holographic and analytical mechanisms may respectively form the neurophysiological foundation of tacit and explicit processing, we shall now briefly consider how these two levels of knowing come to be reciprocally articulated in an individual lifespan.

Tacit and Explicit Levels of Knowing in
Individual Lifespan

An old tenet, widely accepted at the time when embryology was establishing itself as an autonomous discipline, stated that ontogeny formally recapitulates phylogeny. Although the absolute validity of so general and vague a notion can legitimately be doubted, it is undeniable that the development of tacit and explicit knowledge in an individual lifespan offers a number of parallels to the previously suggested evolutionary role of these processes. Thus, adhering to this theme, the following analogies are presented in the sequence in which they unfold.

1. Having occurred more globally in the evolution of human consciousness, tacit processing is undoubtedly the level of knowing that appears first in the course of individual development. Because of the slow unfolding of cognitive growth, infancy and preschool years are primarily characterized by an immediate and global apprehension of oneself and reality in which the capabilities of verbalization, abstraction, and reflexive awareness are absolutely negligible. Corresponding to the evolutionary events that culminated in the specialization of the cerebral hemispheres, is the progressive elaboration of an articulated level of conscious, explicit knowledge within an individual lifespan. This is a slow, gradual process that reaches its highest structural level (i.e., Piagetian formal operations) during early youth and adolescence. Additionally, even in individual development, the gradual attainment of higher semantic levels of information processing is accompanied by a progressive disengagement of the person's thought from the situational "here and now" as well as from the immediacy of his/her experiencing of self.

Therefore, it appears that a primary feature of individual cognitive development is a sort of "temporal gap" between tacit and explicit levels of knowing. On the one hand, the progressive scaffolding of immediate experience occurring throughout infancy, preschool years, and childhood yields a complex system of tacit ordering rules. On the other hand, the slow unfolding of cognitive abilities makes possible awareness, at least in part, of their presence only at a later stage, usually adolescence and early adulthood. Only at this time may the relationship between tacit and explicit knowledge undergo a reorganization, in which the prelogical and emotional apprehensions of the self elaborated thus far can be structured into a conscious self-image capable of actively directing the programming of one's life.

2. As in the course of the evolutionary pathway, a dynamic relationship is established between individual tacit and explicit levels of knowing. Due to this complementarity, deep tacit rules

that supply an individual with the invariant aspects of his/her perception of self and the world, may encounter an unending process of conscious restructuring as a result of the moment-to-moment assimilation of experience.

Nevertheless, it should not be assumed that adulthood represents a sort of "finishing point" in which all the individual tacit ordering processes have been explicated. Tacit and explicit levels of knowing are not regarded as two polarities occupying the extremes of a single continuum, but rather as two independent and irreducible dimensions occurring in constant reciprocal interaction. Because of the irreducibility and oscillative tension between these two dimensions, each individual lifespan is an open-ended, generative process, in which no special state of maturity (i.e., stable equilibrium) is ever reached.

However, corresponding to the evolutionary "choice of the species" that assigned executive control of actions to emergent higher cortical functions, after adolescence the unfolding conscious self-identity similarly becomes the executive regulator of one's interaction with the world.

> We are faced, it seems, with a new problem in analyzing the person. The person is a conglomeration of selves—a sociological entity. Because of our cultural bias toward language and its use, as well as the richness and flexibility that it adds to our existence, the governor of these multiple selves comes to be the verbal system. Indeed, a case can be made that the entire process of maturing in our culture is the process of the verbal system's trying to note and eventually control the behavioral impulses of the many selves that dwell inside us. (Gazzaniga & LeDoux, 1978, p. 161)

Finally, it may be noted that the decentralized control resulting from the opponent and complementary regulation between tacit and explicit knowing might represent, at least in situations involving a certain degree of stress, a sort of tendency toward the disunity of individual consciousness (Marks, 1980; Nagel, 1971; Puccetti, 1981; Tart, 1972, 1980). Although many states of consciousness may to some degree be a function of certain tacit data exerting pressure to be explicated, the possibility of properly decoding them depends on the structure of the conscious self-image in charge—which can be incompatible with the very nature of such tacit data. Therefore, in a systems approach, the unity that a human knowing system usually exhibits is not regarded as an absolute or static entity, but as a *process*—one representing the dynamic and dialectical integration inherent to the coalitional control of a self-organized complexity.

EMOTIONS AND THE PRIMACY
OF PERSONAL MEANING

Assuming that tacit, analogical processes play a crucial role in the scaffolding of the order and regularities with which we are acquainted, it follows that feelings and emotions are primary in personal knowing.

When considered within an evolutionary perspective, the primacy of affect becomes explicit. While cognitive abilities represent one of the final products to emerge from a long evolutionary process, feelings and emotions were probably the first organized knowing system to actively scaffold environmental regularities. Unlike language and cognition, emotional responsiveness is universal among the animal species (Eibl-Eibesfeldt, 1972; Plutchik, 1980; Zajonc, 1980). As a matter of fact, the primary of affective reactions is equally evident in the ontological perspective. From the earliest phases of development and long before they develop anything approximating verbal skills, infants possess both the primary qualities of feelings and the ability to manifest them through expressive motor patterns (Ekman, 1972; Izard, 1977, 1980; Plutchik, 1983).

By nature, however, basic feelings are diffuse, chaotic, and, not easy to decode and control. In order to become specific subjective emotional experiences, feelings have to acquire structural connections with perceptions and actions. In other words, an emotion is an internal process of control acquired by structuring a relationship (i.e., a schema) between feelings, perceptions, and motor patterns in memory representation (Giblin, 1981; Pribram, 1967, 1971, 1980c).

Therefore, emotions should be regarded as organized, complex experiences whose dynamic unity may be understood only as one proceeds toward more integrated levels of systemic coherence. Within this perspective, the notion of "emotional schemata" introduced by Leventhal (1979, 1980) and other similar concepts (Bower, 1981; Lang, 1979) represent promising, integrative models that attempt to account for the correlations among the many components of emotional experience (e.g., perception, imagery, memory, etc.). The essential feature of the emotional schemata model is the relevance given to an analogical memory mechanism believed to be active during emotional processing and composed of images constructed from the key perceptual features of emotion-eliciting situations and the visceral, motor, and expressive patterns that accompany these situations. Thus, emotional schemata are structural configurations in memory representation that act as a pattern against which the ongoing sensory inflow is compared and made meaningful.

As we will see, such integrating models may offer a useful theoretical framework for the understanding of the development of emotional differentiation and personal meaning.

Development of Emotional Differentiation

The notion of "emotional schemata" is an effective conceptual device for explaining the progressive integration, occurring in the course of development, between inborn patterns of emotional reactions and acquired emotional differentiation. While the ontogenesis of basic feelings is primarily a function of the unfolding of maturational stages (a rather aspecific and impersonal process), developmental experiences determine the structures (emotional schemata) in which these basic feelings will be scaffolded and assigned highly specific and personal emotional tonalities.

The fact that a schema is essentially a neural configuration acting as a pattern for the comparison of impulses permits us to look at emotional differentiation as an ongoing matching process between preformed emotional schemata and incoming feelings. The search for congruity (pattern recognition) would act as the main regulator, giving functional continuity to the temporal progression of the whole process.

Given the rather slow progression of cognitive abilities, the emergence of differentiated patterns of self-perception and self-consciousness will be primarily a function of the basic ensembles of emotional schemata that provide direction and focus to the unfolding perceptual–cognitive processes (Izard, 1980; Izard & Buechler, 1980, 1983). Emotional schemata, acting as "criterion images" for subsequent match-to-pattern processes, predispose available cognitive abilities toward the selection of specific domains of exchange in the interaction with the world. Thus, through the structuring of knowledge contents coherent with one's immediate apprehension of self, the ongoing assembling of emotional schemata provides an essential continuity and unitarity to the development of conscious experience.

Personal Meaning

Although Bartlett (1932) proposed that the human scaffolding of experience is primarily an "effort after meaning," only within the last decade has the problem of meaning been recognized as central to cognitive psychology. Specifically, the interconnection between meaning and tacit processing has become more evident (Mahoney, 1982; Van Den Bergh & Eelen, 1984), as well described by Weimer (1974):

> I would like to argue that the entire problem of tacit knowledge is nothing more, nothing less, than the problem of meaning. In this sense, there is only one problem that has ever existed in psychology, and everything the field has investigated is merely a manifestation of that problem, a different aspect of the same elephant, an elephant that we have grasped at since the dawn of reflective thought without ever reaching at all. (p. 428)

Furthermore, within a perspective in which the mind is looked upon as a motor system whose self-referential nature is articulated in a coherent and unitary organization and reorganization of its classificatory activity, "meaning" becomes the underlying interrelationship of all "higher" mental processes, manifested in each such process but not identifiable with any of them. Thus meaning is always context dependent: dependent upon the framework that relates all "higher" mental processes" (Weimer, 1977, p. 297).

In view of what has been said up to this point, how can this unitary framework be summarized? Unequivocally, the progressive hierarchical organization of differentiated ensembles of emotional schemata is what provides the individual's tacit level of processing an organizational unity that makes every aspect of mental processing highly personal and idiosyncratic. In perception, attention, remembering, and understanding, the continuous emotional modulation (deriving from the matching between ordered patterns of emotional schemata and ongoing experience) provides a tacit apperceptive scaffolding that delimits the kinds of experiences one may expect and seek at the conscious level of interaction with the world. Finally, the sense of uniqueness and oneness, correlated to the continuity of personal meaning processes, is also based on the organizational unity of one's emotional domain. In fact, the highly personal arrangement of one's emotional schemata is what provides the decoding context that enables one to recognize and experience a wide variety of ongoing inner states within a single coherent and continuous dimension.

NOTES

1. Evolutionary knowledge constraints are not to be regarded as absolute or fixed entities, as was the case for traditional perspectives referring to innatism. Indeed, if knowledge processes are emergent, interactive products of the ongoing match between the knowing subject and reality, then knowledge itself appears to be far removed from a mere sensorial copy of external reality (empiricism), as well as from a mere unfolding of structures already preformed in the individual (innatism). A systems approach, therefore, entails an interactionistic perspective, in which internal and external variables are intertwined in an opponent regulation process. In simpler terms, even if knowledge constraints are the product of a long evolutionary process of exploration and experimentation, they require further ontological exploration and experimentation to become effective computational devices. That is, *knowledge constraints become knowledge structures only through the scaffolding of experience.*

2. Previous research, currently receiving renewed attention, has shown that mental processes are consistently accompanied by electromyographic (EMG) activity, though too weak to activate overt motor behavior (Max, 1937; Jacobson, 1932, quoted by Van Den Bergh & Eelen, 1984). Van Den Bergh and Eelen (1984) reported that recent research has confirmed those earlier findings; for example, the findings that silent reading produces motor activity in speech muscles (McGuigan, 1970), or that thoughts with affective content are accompanied by specific types of EMG patterns of the face muscles (Cacioppo & Petty, 1981; Sirota & Schwartz, 1982).

CHAPTER THREE

SOME GENERAL REMARKS ON SELFHOOD PROCESSES, ATTACHMENT, AND IDENTITY

SELFHOOD AS A DIALECTICAL, INTERACTIVE PROCESS

The self is not something fixed inside my head. If it exists at all, my
self is a process: the unending process by which I turn new
experience into knowledge.—Bronowski (1971)

A distinctive feature of the human knowing system is its ability
to actively build its own identity through a progressive differentiation
between self and nonself. Furthermore, while the nonself may
theoretically be divided into social and nonsocial domains, the
selection of the social domain as a basis for comparison suggests
that an essential component of the self-differentiation process is
the *similarity* between perceiver and perceived (Hamlyn, 1974; Lewis
& Brooks-Gunn, 1979).

In addition to being the underlying epistemological basis of
self-referential activity, the need for similarity between perceiver
and perceived logically implies that any self-knowledge has its
foundation in the presence of, and interaction with, others. The
well-known theory that human beings acquire self-knowledge
through interaction with other people—the "looking-glass self"
(Cooley, 1902; Mead, 1934)—is at present supported by increasing
evidence coming mainly from research on primates (Gallup, 1977;
Hayes & Nissen, 1971; Linden, 1974). In particular, studies of self-
recognition processes using the mirror-image stimulation with primates have shown that prior exposure to interactions with others
is a fundamental requisite for any rudimentary form of self-rec-

ognition (Gallup, 1970; Gallup & McClure, 1971; Gallup, McClure, Hill, & Bundy, 1971).[1]

Although such patterns and processes are infinitely more rudimentary than those in humans, even in primates the ability to perform self-recognition seems to be the emergent product of a dynamic interplay among opponent processes. On one hand, others provide the template that permits the scaffolding of a unitary perception of self, but on the other hand, it is as if this unitary perception of self can only be experienced and recognized through an active demarcation from the perceived other.

The fact that a stable opponent interaction between self and others is an essential requisite for the acquisition of elementary patterns of self-recognition reveals that such a process is not only a self-referent, cognitive procedure, but also represents an ontological demarcation that reflects the irreducible duality of our sensory experience—that is, the distinction between self-perception (inner sense) and world-perception (outer sense). The ability to experience oneself both as subject and object—an undeniable as well as puzzling hallmark of our sense of self—most certainly stems from this duality of sensory experience (Morin, 1981; Varela, 1979).

Therefore, from the earliest stages of development, every human knowing system actively integrates two flows of stimuli that are distinct but always simultaneous: self-perception and perception of the world. Thus, any information about the outside world inevitably corresponds to information about the self and, conversely, self-knowledge development parallels the process by which the individual comes to understand external reality. In this way the elaboration of knowledge appears to be a *unitary* process that occurs through a dynamic interplay of two polarities, the self and the world, that can be metaphorically equated to the two sides of a coin: A subject's self-knowledge always involves his or her conception of reality, and conversely, every conception of reality is directly connected to the subject's view of self (Bronowski, 1971; Churchland, 1984; Dennett, 1978).

ATTACHMENT PROCESSES AND SELF-IDENTITY

Just as we learn to see ourselves in a mirror, so the child becomes conscious of himself by seeing his reflection in the mirror of other people's consciousness of himself. —Popper (1977)

As a logical consequence of the assumption that human knowledge is imbued with interactive–reflective properties, a crucial role is attributed to interpersonal and relational domains in the development of self-identity. I therefore agree with Ainsworth, Blehar, Waters, and Wall (1978) in considering attachment theory (Bowlby, 1969, 1973, 1980a, 1983) as a sort of explanatory hypothesis supplying a structured framework for understanding and organizing the available observational and experimental data, that is, a new, integrating paradigm of human development that gives us an inclusive and organized view of the dominant factors that contribute to the structuring of self-knowledge.

Indeed, from an evolutionary perspective, it is clear that prolonged dependent and emotionally charged relationships with others parallels the increase in complexity of the human mind. In other words the gradual attainment of a sense of identity and personal agency requires a stable interpersonal context throughout development. Thus, attachment processes and self-organizing abilities are integrally interwoven; the progressive development of familial patterns of attachment represents the key decoding context that provides focus and direction to the child's unfolding cognitive–emotional abilities. Beginning with mere physical bonds in early infancy, attachment becomes a highly structured vehicle through which increasingly complex and unlimited information about oneself and the world become available. The crucial role that attachment plays in the development of self-knowledge may best be summarized in Bowlby's own words:

> A young child's experience of an encouraging, supportive and co-operative mother, and a little later father, gives him a sense of worth, a belief in the helpfulness of others, and a favourable model on which to build future relationships. Furthermore, by enabling him to explore his environment with confidence and to deal with it effectively, such experience also promotes his sense of competence. Thenceforward, provided family relationships continue favourable, not only do these early patterns of thought, feeling and behavior persist, but personality becomes increasingly structured to operate in moderately controlled and resilient ways, and increasingly capable of continuing so despite adverse circumstances. (1983, p. 378)

In the course of human development, attachment plays somewhat of a differential role. During the formative years, attachment processes exert a profound influence on identity development and self-knowledge formation. Throughout adulthood, affective social ties contribute to the maintenance and stabilization of acquired selfhood structures and similarly allow for the integration of more complex levels of knowledge.

Attention will now be given to the mechanisms underlying the close interdependence between attachment and selfhood processes in each of the developmental periods.

Attachment and Identity Development

The unifying thread of identity development is the progressive emergence of an actor's sense of uniqueness and oneness acquired from the knowledge that self is different from others and has its own attributes. Because of the slow unfolding of cognitive abilities, children acquire such knowledge long before they are able to reflect upon it and are not able to transform this tacit and immediate apprehension of themselves into a full sense of personal identity until they enter adolescence.

Within a systems approach, it is of paramount importance to understand the development of selfhood as a coherent whole, rather than to focus on limited aspects of emotional differentiation and cognitive growth. Adopting this perspective clarifies the crucial developmental role that a primary and exclusive bond with only one or two specific people may play. Indeed, evidence from several sources shows how difficult it is for children to form a secure attachment with more than one person because attachment figures tend to be arranged in a hierarchical order with the principal figure at the top (Bowlby, 1969, 1983; Parkes & Stevenson-Hinde, 1982).

Uniqueness, therefore, seems to be a basic factor in developing attachment relationships. A unique relationship with an attachment figure, yields a sort of template within which otherwise fragmentary information about self and the world can be organized into a coherent whole. In other words, uniqueness of primary bonds seems to be a necessary condition for perceiving and recognizing our wholeness, and may function in a manner analogous to the principles of organization that underlie a conceptual structure of understanding (Marris, 1982). Furthermore, at least during early development, when cognition is more or less closely bound to the existing situation, children can abstract their own sense of personal uniqueness from the very experience of being involved in a unique relationship. In other words, building a unique relationship with a significant other represents an important way (perhaps not only during maturational stages) one may obtain a sense of uniqueness and oneness.

Within this kind of emotional relationship, how can the learning processes of the child be outlined? Because knowing is essentially a self-referent matching process, imitation and modeling (Bandura, 1969, 1985) are at the very core of learning and development. If, in order to understand a child's developing wholeness, we assume a unitarian point of view, imitation and modeling should be considered at the corresponding level of systemic self-reference, that is to say, as nothing else than *identification processes*. The definition of the term "identification" is somewhat debatable and many clinicians unsympathetic toward the psychoanalytic approach prefer not to use it at all. Nevertheless, it is a rather common observation in clinical practice that children and adolescents frequently exhibit behavioral and cognitive styles that can easily be recognized as similar to those of their parents. Thus, it is perhaps preferable to maintain the term "identification" since it shares the same root as "identity" and is therefore appropriate to indicate a match-to-pattern process leading to the latter.

We will now briefly examine how identification processes can be viewed within the continuous dynamic interplay between self and others. At any point during the developmental process a child's ongoing sense of self can be seen as the emergent product of two opposite tendencies: one outward and the other inward.

Initially, the self is undifferentiated and faces a world just as confusing and unintelligible as itself. The capacity to recognize relevant information about oneself through the perceived similarity between one's ongoing self-perception and the perception of a significant other (identification processes) appears to be a function of a general "outward tendency." On the other hand, the elaboration of a genuine sense of self also requires a turning away from the source of identification. This "inward tendency" involves the ability to transform the perceived similarity to an attachment figure into a stable personal attribute (identity processes). In other words, children imitate the roles and attitudes of their attachment figures, but, in the process, make them their own, creating a single, subjectively coherent personal identity (Hoffman, 1971, 1975, 1978).

Identification processes appear to be connected with different mechanisms and effects depending upon the particular developmental period under consideration. In infancy the reciprocal interplay between child and caregiver has a pervasive influence on the structuring of fundamental emotions and, consequently, on the first stable patterns of self-perception. Through regularities drawn from caregivers' behaviors and motivations, the infant can start to connect diffuse basic feelings with specific perceptions, actions, and memories, turning them into specific subjective emotional experiences, that is, emotional schemata.

Later on, in preschool years and in childhood, because of their limited cognitive abilities, children's identification processes are primarily mediated by the immediate emotional aspects of the ongoing significant attachment relationship. These features continue to play a predominant role in the child's emotional differentiation as well as on the structuring of a rather stable and enduring sense of self.

In adolescence, the emergence of logical/deductive abilities shifts identification processes toward the internalization of highly abstract life values and existential axioms taken from a significant attachment figure. However, whether or not higher semantic levels of information processing are available, it is quite evident that identification, just as any complex abstract ordering, is mainly a tacit process. As Musil noted years ago in his masterpiece *The Man Without Qualities* (1979), adolescents and youths usually consider the values of their parents to be ridiculous or boring, only to discover later on in life, and often quite suddenly, that they have nevertheless acquired them and are behaving in accordance with them.

In summary, throughout the developmental stages characterized by unfolding cognitive growth and emotional differentiation, patterns of attachment shift from the lability typical of early infancy to the stability of adolescence and youth. Concurrently, the reciprocal interplay between identification and identity processes becomes increasingly complex and articulated, enabling developing youngsters to form an even more comprehensive view of themselves and the world with which they can begin to actively structure their life planning.

Attachment and Selfhood Processes in Adulthood

As the "cognitive revolution" takes place in adolescence and youth, attachment, although shifting toward a more abstract level, maintains its fundamental interdependence with selfhood processes and personal meaning. Because attachment to significant others is central to the structuring of self-knowledge throughout the course of development, during adulthood new kinds of attachment emerge (e.g., intimate, love relationships) that acquire the function of confirming, supporting, and further expanding personal reality.

Studies on personal loss and bereavement provide widespread support for the crucial role that an important affectional bond plays in the preservation of one's sense of identity. Such research suggests that grief may be conceptualized as an interruption in personal meaning, and that the grieving process ends only when an individual has restructured his/her sense of self (Bowlby, 1980a; Marris, 1982; Parkes, 1972). From this perspective, an attachment style is viewed as a self-referent process aimed at preserving an individual's systemic coherence through the ongoing production of emotional experiences in keeping with his/her perceived personal meaning.

Of course, not all kinds of affectional bonds can be regarded as attachments in the sense that I have just described. For example, Weiss (1982) found that only individuals who had recently become divorced reported states of emotional distress that could not be soothed by friendships and were generally characterized as "loneliness."[2] Therefore, only certain kinds of long-lived, face-to-face relationships with an appreciable level of emotional intimacy are able to bring remarkable stabilizing effects on one's sense of identity, and they are usually few in number even over the course of a lifetime. In other words, although it takes different forms, the same interdependence between unique attachments and stability of selfhood found in prior developmental stages exists in adulthood as well. This is understandable if we consider that the involvement in unique relationships begins early in life, and adult bonds of love seem to grow out of those very first attachments (Marris, 1982).

Therefore, if the continuity and systemic coherence of personal meaning processes rest on a balanced interplay between the individual and his/her personal network of unique relationships, we may then reasonably suppose that the most disrupting emotions a person can ever experience in life are those elicited in the course of establishing, maintaining, and breaking such relationships. Life-events studies carried out within this perspective show that numerous life crises are related to losses or alterations of significant bonds, and therefore support the idea that an alteration of one's affective balance is an important moderating variable involved in the production of emotional disorders commonly called neurotic disturbances (Bowlby, 1977a; Brown, 1982; Brown & Harris, 1978; Henderson, 1982; Henderson, Byrne, & Duncan-Jones, 1981).

In summary, with the emergence of a full sense of personhood, by now stable and differentiated, the interdependence between self and others (i.e., between our simultaneous experiencing ourselves as subjects and objects) actually shifts toward a more abstract level of interaction. During any period of lifespan development, our ongoing sense of identity may be regarded as the emergent product of a dynamic balance between an outward tendency to perceive our being a part of the whole, and an inward tendency to perceive the wholeness of our being a part (Sameroff, 1982). This means that even in adulthood, though with greater abstraction, selfhood is made recognizable and decodable to itself only through interactions with others. This is because any category applied to oneself is also applied in understanding others, and conversely, any category discovered in others at once becomes recognizable and applicable to the self. In short, accepting the broader implication of the statement that self-knowledge relies on others is equivalent to acknowledging the epistemic character of attachment processes. This implies that the continuous interplay with others' experiences—either in a direct or a symbolic way—is the basic process that transforms the lifespan development of reflective selfhood into a spiraling, open-ended process.

> Man is a machine by birth but a self by experience. And the special character of the self lies in its experience not of nature but of others. A man enters the lives of other men more directly than he can enter nature, because he recognizes his own thoughts and feelings in them; he learns to make theirs his own, and to find in himself a deeper self that has the features of all humanity. The knowledge of nature teaches him to act, and makes him master of the creation. The knowledge of self does not teach him to act but to be; it steeps him in the human predicament and predicament of life; it makes him one with all the creatures. (Bronowski, 1971, p. 114)

NOTES

1. An interesting remark is that the ability to differentiate between self and others, and thus to accomplish self-recognition, seems to be a specific property exhibited,

though to different degrees, only by great apes and man. This suggests that such an ability surfaces in the evolutionary scale only when a certain level of self-organized complexity is achieved. In addition, more than being a mere result of cumulative learning, this property signals the emergence of a new organized level of self-reference, namely "reflexive self-reference."

> The capacity for self-recognition, although influenced by learning, is predicated on a sense of identity. The unique feature of mirror-image stimulation is that the identity of the observer and his reflection in a mirror are necessarily one and the same. The capacity to correctly infer the identity of the reflection must, therefore, presuppose an already existent identity on the part of the organism making this inference. Without an identity of your own it would be impossible to recognize yourself. (Gallup, 1977, p. 334)

2. In a lifespan attachment perspective, symptoms of loneliness appear to be very similar and overlap those of separation distress. As Weiss (1982) noted, however, separation distress is caused by the actual loss of a significant person and the desperate desire to have him/her back, whereas in loneliness, the individual experiences pervasive barrenness and emptiness. Therefore, loneliness is apparently a separation distress that has no object and may probably be ascribed to a perceived lack of emotional intimacy in ongoing relationships. Other theoretical and methodological approaches to loneliness are found in Peplau and Perlman (1982).

PART TWO

DEVELOPMENTAL AND
ORGANIZATIONAL MODELS

CHAPTER FOUR

DEVELOPMENT

How a system establishes its identity (its autonomy) correlates with
how it generates information; the mechanisms of identity are
interwoven with the mechanisms of knowledge. —Varela (1979)

INTRODUCTORY REMARKS

Because attachment processes and self-nonself differentiation are
so closely correlated, the parent–child (P-C) relationship can be
regarded as the foundation underlying both (1) the development
of identity and attitude toward oneself and (2) the development
of interpersonal behavior and attitude toward reality. The crucial
role of the P-C relationship depends basically on certain structural
characteristics that make it distinctly different from all adult–adult
relationships to which it gives rise. These unique features are summarized below.

1. The difference in cognitive abilities between parents and
children is greater than in all other human relationships. This
difference makes the emotional bonds with parents unique in each
person's life, precisely because none of us could possibly have had
any point of reference to compare them to anything else. As a
result, the developmental identification processes differ from those
that characterize adulthood. The child does not internalize the
world of people who are meaningful to him/her as one of the
possible worlds, but as *the* world, the only one that exists and
the only conceivable one. Complementarity, therefore, is a hallmark
of the P-C relationship even though, as we shall see, it may take
on a variety of forms and contents, depending upon the specific
pattern of family interaction and the particular developmental stage
of the child.

2. The rate of change in P-C interaction is greater than in all
other human relationships. Paralleling the steplike attainment of

higher semantic levels of information processing, the interactional patterns and the domains of exchange of the P-C relationship are constantly changing in response to the child's "discoveries" and initiatives. Therefore, the search for autonomy may be regarded as another basic dimension of the P-C relationship. As Hinde (1979) argued, many developmental events may best be regarded as children's attempts to redefine their role in the ongoing relationship with parents.

Thus, once again we encounter an instance of an opponent regulation process: the complementarity of the P-C relationship undergoing rhythmic differentiation through the continuous interplay with the search for autonomy. Only by the end of adolescence, when a full sense of personhood emerges, will the individual have acquired a stable and well-defined autonomy with respect to attachment figures. In a nutshell, the interplay between complementarity and the search for autonomy represents an explication, at an *explicit* level, of the parallel differentiation between self and others that is being carried out at a *tacit* level.

Finally, because our essential focus should be the understanding of how the whole coherence of a developing child is achieved and maintained (Sander, 1975; Sroufe, 1979) and since "embeddedness" (e.g., any level of analysis is intertwined with the others) is a basic feature of any complex system (Lerner & Busch-Rossnagel, 1981;

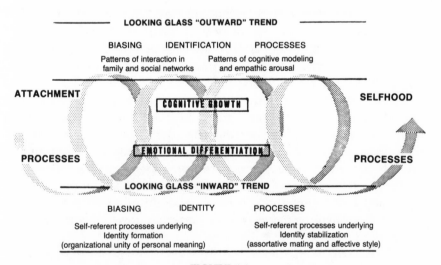

FIGURE 4-1.

Lerner *et al.*, 1980), an adequate description of development should be unitary. It should, in other words, illustrate the progressive integration of attachment processes, developing self-knowledge, cognitive growth, and emotional differentiation while taking into account the family and environmental variables that influence the entire process. In short, seen as a whole, it should look very much like the diagram shown in Figure 4-1.

With this intent, we will now examine the development of selfhood processes through the stages that characterize them most: Infancy and preschool years (from birth to about 5–6 years of age), childhood (roughly corresponding to 6–12 years of age) and adolescence and youth (from about 12–18 years of age).

INFANCY AND PRESCHOOL YEARS

Self-Recognition

During the 1st and 2nd years of life, the available cognitive processes are syncretic and made up of sensorimotor schemata blended with basic feelings and imaginal representations. The attention span is narrow and the child, only capable of centering on part of the immediate situation, constantly shifts his/her focus of attention among the available features of that situation.

The primary feature of early cognition involves the child's inability to fully differentiate his/her own self from the environment. Infants are considerably self-centered in regard to their own representations and feelings; they do not pay much attention to external reality but assimilate it into global undifferentiated schemata. In short, they have a "subject-bound" attitude (Strauss & Lewin, 1981).

Infants, however, are not to be regarded as cognitively inept. Their cognitive abilities are considerably greater than is traditionally believed. It was probably because of the adherence to a sensory, "passive" theory of mind, that it has taken so long to acknowledge their existence (Forman, 1982; Gelman, 1979).

Evidence suggests that cognitive developments during this period are basically independent of linguistic developments. This lends support to the hypothesis that language is not an initiating cause of conceptual transformation,[1] but rather considerably facilitates the further expansion of conceptual development once it has been initiated by infants' ordering of their sensorimotor schemata (Langer, 1981, 1982). As a consequence, the first 2 years of life are the time when the basic requisites for the further development of self-knowledge are established: A sense of self becomes separated from the perception of others, who, in turn, come to be perceived as physical entities to whom one's own characteristics are attributed.

Paraphrasing experimental mirror-image situations, parenting behavior can be considered to work as a sort of mirror-analogous device in human self-recognition processes. In other words, the behaviors of caregivers operate as a mirror held up to an infant through which is reflected to him/her a sense of self. This sense does not remain a mere sensorial datum, but rather directs and coordinates self-recognition patterns until the infant becomes able to perceive him/herself consistently with that sense.

Through what processes does the "looking-glass effect" take place during this very early period? Studies on the mother–infant dyad show that the synchrony and congruency of their responses in interaction are regarded as the infant's essential source of meaningful information (Lewis & Rosenblum, 1974). The rhythmic interdependence between infants and their caregivers seems to be at the very root of their attachment as well as of communication, and the infant learns to control its environment by developing a contingency analysis of their interaction (Brazelton, 1983; Brazelton, Koslowski, & Main, 1974; Levine, 1982; Schaffer & Crook, 1980; Stern, 1974). Emerging contingency patterns, in turn, facilitate further development of a sense of self by structuring a basic self-referent loop: a cyclical reverberation of basic feelings around the approach–avoidance oscillative equilibrium reached in the P-C relationship.[2]

Only when this sense of self is integrated with the developing sense of permanence and continuity in time (e.g., the Piagetian stage of object permanence) is *self-recognition* generally achieved. Self-recognition does not evolve in a simple, unitary manner, but requires the development of many skills that the infant must integrate into a true sense of self, usually within the 2nd year of life (Bertenthal & Fischer, 1978).

It should be stressed that recognition of the self consists not only of a "cognitive" demarcation between self and nonself, but also involves an emotional attitude toward the nonself—a kind of "feeling tone" about the social world, similar to Erikson's (1963) concept of "basic trust." Roughly, this basic feeling tone corresponds to emotional schemata that convey the information that the social world is more or less reliable or the expectation of how satisfactorily one's needs will be met. The principle factor that determines the quality of this feeling tone is, of course, the quality of the caregivers' response to the infant. Particularly during the early period of life, the more their parents offer an atmosphere of unconditioned acceptance beyond the necessary care and protection, the more infants will acquire a feeling that the world and the people in it are reliable.

Finally, self-recognition patterns represent the basis for future learning, supplying a set of basic tacit rules that enable the child (with the aid of emerging linguistic abilities) to further elaborate the invariant structures upon which his/her perception of self and others depend.

Parent–Child Relationship

With a more stable sense of self and the unfolding of new cognitive abilities, children are now able to more and more actively influence the interactions with their caregivers. The conceptualization gradually emancipates itself from global, undifferentiated emotional reactions and physiological patterns, and children become more capable of accommodating themselves to environmental data. The attention span widens and sensorimotor–affective–imaginative cognition is replaced by a perceptual cognition that permits affective and imaginative processes to be increasingly linked to key perceptual features of the environment. However, because perception, by its nature, depends on the ongoing stimulus flow, children cannot detach themselves from the external situation and its influence— for example, they have an "object-bound" attitude (Strauss & Lewin, 1981).

This infantile "realism" makes the emotional bonds between parents and children idiosyncratic. Indeed, the infant's early relationship with his/her parents is absolutely unique. On the one hand, infants have a compulsory need for contact, affection, and protection. On the other hand, they will not be able to depict an alternative relationship to the one that historical contingencies have imposed upon them. Under such conditions, the child's identification with parents, rather than a question of choice, is a "must" that occurs in an entirely tacit, automatic way (Berger & Luckmann, 1966).

In addition to their crucial role in determining what information on self and the world is significant and how it will be processed, parents themselves provide the most meaningful sources of information for the child's elaboration of a sense of self.

1. One set of significant information comes from the affective components of parents' attachment to their children. Within a good reciprocal attachment, children come to perceive themselves as lovable and competent, that is, capable of controlling a reliable interpersonal environment that fosters expected outcomes. They are confident and effusive in their attachment patterns. Conversely, if the reciprocity of attachment is poor, children are more likely to perceive themselves as unlovable and incompetent, that is, more or less disarmed in the hands of an uncontrollable and unreliable environment. Such patterns of attachment engender avoidant, aggressive and/or ambivalent behaviors (Ainsworth, 1979; Main & Weston, 1982).

2. A second set of significant information is derived from the way parents either facilitate or interfere with a child's search for autonomy. The early search for autonomy is characterized by the child's initiating temporary separations from caregivers, autonomous explorations, and by the tendency to self-mastering and independence. At this stage, the problem for children to resolve is the struggle between being controlled by outsiders and of learning controls for themselves (Brazelton, 1974). Parents' implicit and explicit reactions to the child's initiatives and their availability as a "safe base" for his/her explorations are of the utmost importance. Of course, a good relationship with both parents, and a high degree of exchange and coordination among the parents themselves, will certainly produce the best effects for a genuine sense of competence and autonomy. Main and Weston (1981) reported that children with a secure relationship with both parents are the most confident and competent; children who do not have a secure relationship with either parent are less confident and competent, while those who have established a secure relationship with only one parent tend to fall in the middle.

The Emergence of Emotions and Consciousness

From the earliest phases of development, the infant is equipped with both basic feelings and the ability to communicate them through expressive motor mechanisms (Eibl-Eibesfeldt, 1972, 1979; Ekman, 1972, Izard, 1977, 1980). The quality of early caregiver–infant reciprocity is an essential source of cues for scaffolding basic feelings into fundamental, discrete emotions through the linkages these feelings progressively acquire with perception, imagination, and motor activity.

However, without a rudimentary self-knowledge, an emotion-eliciting stimulus may produce an emotional expression but not an emotional experience (Lewis & Brooks-Gunn, 1979). Only during the 2nd year, because of the development of a rather stable self-recognition, does the child become able to localize feeling tones and fundamental emotions within the self, organizing them as prototypical emotional experiences. A clear example of this is the fear of strangers and of separation from caregivers exhibited by children in their 2nd year of life, which parallels the emergence of an increased awareness of the distinctness of self from others (Wolf, 1982).

Since perceiving another person's affective state is a necessary condition for recognizing the same feeling within the self, patterns of attachment and identification processes are the unitary framework through which emotional differentiation unfolds during the entire preschool-years period. Thus, fundamental emotions more complex than fear, such as shame or guilt, can be experienced only after the 2nd year, when children can better internalize the standards of their caregivers. In other words, while the ontogenesis of fundamental emotions is predominantly a function of maturational stages, the child, through identification processes and cognitive growth, scaffolds these emotions into an even more unitary and coherent pattern of self-perception and self-evaluation. Let us now examine the essential aspects of this process, which becomes relatively stabilized only around the end of preschool years.

Infantile consciousness is truly affective in nature and quality. Thus, the sense of self is primarily organized around prototypical emotional schemata whose ordering, in turn, depends on the specific quality of ongoing patterns of attachment (Izard & Buechler, 1980).

These basic emotional schemata provide the key perceptual–affective features for assimilating ongoing experience; and since internal language is hardly used, for the child they come to represent absolute reality.

According to Tomkins (1978), "this postulated set of innate linkages between stimulus, affect and response suggests that human beings are to some extent innately endowed with the possibility of organized if primitive scenes or happenings somewhat under their own control beginning as early as the neonatal period" (p. 211). Therefore, a scene represents the basic unit of analysis from the viewpoint of a child's experiencing of life—an ensemble of emotional schemata that rehearse and reproduce a sense of self out of a prior concrete experience.

It follows that the most intense affect-laden scenes will function as "criterion images," which influence available cognitive abilities by integrating them with other scenes on the basis of analogy rather than by mere similarity of detail. This analogical differentiation, or, in Tomkins's (1978) terms this "psychological magnification," is extremely important in maximizing the coherence of unfolding patterns of self-perception, since previous scenes are connected with presently experienced as well as anticipated ones.

> Psychological magnification begins, then, in earliest infancy when the infant imagines, via co-assembly, a possible improvement in what is already a rewarding scene, attempts to do what may be necessary to bring it about, and so produces and connects a set of scenes which continue to reward him food, and its excitement and enjoyment, and also with the excitement and enjoyment of remaking the world closer to the heart's desire. He is doing what he will continue to try to do all his life—to command the scenes he wishes to play. Like Charlie Chaplin, he will try to write, direct, produce, criticize, and promote the scenes in which he casts himself as hero. (pp. 214–215)

Therefore, during infancy and preschool years, several ensembles of scenes, hierarchically ordered around the most affect-laden ones, become differentiated in parallel. Around the end of the preschool years, when the basic set of prototypic significant scenes has become sufficiently differentiated, amplified, and magnified to foster an initial rudimentary conceptualization, a raw draft of the "nuclear scene" (Tomkins, 1978) becomes available, and self-perception patterns, in turn, become rather stable and capable of anticipating the immediate future.

It should be specified that, in order for a nuclear scene to be formed, a single, "primary" experience is not enough, since the effects of one isolated experience, whatever its quality, fade with the passing of time. A nuclear scene originates from an affect-laden situation that becomes prototypical as a consequence of its being repeatedly experienced by the child in situations that, though similar, are not exactly identical, and that he/she experiences, not so much out of conscious intention, but because of an inability to avoid them.

The formalization of a nuclear scene consists in ordering the different ensembles of scenes into a recurrent loop that oscillates between two main clusters of prototypical emotional schemata selected and differentiated through early attachment patterns. It basically represents a "minimum" of a self-maintaining cognitive organization that through the cyclic and recursive interplay of its opponent processes is capable of simultaneously generating one's own pattern of self-perception and a whole ordered sequence of behaviors and emotions.

For instance, consider a child who, having repeatedly experienced separation, loss, and/or rejection, has a nuclear scene that oscillates between helplessness/sadness on one side and anger on the other. On the one hand, he/she is endowed with a rather differentiated self-perception centered around a sense of detachment from others, whether it is perceived in a passive or imposed way (helplessness), or in an active, self-produced way (anger and aggressiveness). On the other hand, the opponent regulation process prevents withdrawal and the experience of loneliness (connected to helplessness) from going beyond critical limits, due to the opponent activation of outward, contact-seeking behavior (connected to anger). This feeling, in turn, is generally prevented from going beyond critical limits—and producing still more separations and rejections—by the activation of the opponent process that restores withdrawal and recentering on the self.

It should be stressed that the cyclic interplay between opponent boundaries is *internal* to the infant and makes no reference to the environment. It is as though contact itself arouses anger and withdrawal, and withdrawal leads again to contact that leads again to anger and withdrawal. Hence, the emergence of stable patterns of self-perception from the interplay of emotional and cognitive factors can be regarded as a rhythmic differentiation of opponent processes that fluctuate between extreme boundaries of meaning (Weimer, 1983).

Finally, from this perspective, the preschool-years differentiation of individual nuclear scenes underlies the further development of individual differences in normal personality, and even more significantly, in abnormal personality (Abelson, 1981). Although for each child there are relatively few nuclear scenes, the rate and continuity of their growth is an important variable since nuclear scenes provide direction and focus to cognitive processes by selecting specific domains of experience, thereby influencing the content that knowledge itself will assume.

Selfhood Processes in Preschool Years

Around the 4th or 5th year, a remarkable rearrangement of the sense of self takes place due to increasing interplay between emotional differentiation (amplification of nuclear scenes) and cognitive growth (conceptual perspective taking).

The acquisition of a sense that others are "intentional persons" (and therefore, sources of feelings, thoughts, and plans separate from one's own), coupled with the inherent increase in decentering and distancing abilities, yields a further differentiation between self and nonself. This, in turn, allows the child to perceive him/ herself as a rather independent agency (Wolf, 1982). Moreover, since the emotion-articulating mechanisms underlying identification processes depend on the child's sense of other, he/she can now detect more subtle cues for recognizing emotions, which creates a greater sense of autonomy.

The formalized nuclear scenes, therefore, are no longer perceived as emotional *states* that intrude upon the mind of the subject but as emotional *experiences* for the child to act upon. For example, the separation distress that emerged at the time of self-recognition rapidly fades away with age; and at 4 to 5 years of age, most children maintain exploratory play throughout the separation episodes without apparent distress. Children no longer need to find security only through physical contact, for they are capable of elaborating and maintaining a shared set of plans and goals with their caregiver even when the person is temporarily absent. Of course, the capacity to have such integrated plans depends on the degree and quality of reciprocity of attachment patterns. Children abused by their parents, for example, are low on conceptual perspective taking, and therefore experience an object-bound attitude and separation distress until much later in development.

> It is clear, therefore, that a mother who usually takes account of her child's perspective and interests is likely to have a child who reciprocates by taking account of his mother's perspective and interests—yet another example of the powerful influence of a parent and, also, we may assume, of learning from a model. (Bowlby, 1983, p. 369)

The preschooler's sense of identity, which is continuously reelaborated on an affective/prelogical level, will be expressed mostly by the way children enact their sense of self. This is revealed not only in their affective relationships, but also through games, fantasies, and fairy tales in which they identify with their favorite characters. It is primarily through understanding children's attitude toward reality that a discerning observer can reconstruct the developing knowledge of self and world. A clinical vignette can perhaps exemplify this point.

Eric, age 40, a severely depressed journalist, at the beginning of therapy could not remember much of his personal history, and had almost no memories of his infancy and childhood. With some effort, he was able to recall a tangle of images and sensations concerning the birth of his younger brother when he was 5 years old. Eric's parents were rich and could afford to carry on an active social life by hiring nurses and housemaids to care for their small children. Images depicted him sneaking into his parents' bedroom while they were out for social engagements and when the nurse could not see him, in order to lull his little brother. Accompanying him in the darkness of the night, while he sat beside the cradle, wrapped in a blanket for protection, were sensations of dejection and coldness.

This recollection permits us to reconstruct what was probably Eric's sense of identity at that age. The distinct sense of loneliness and separation from the parents was no longer inferred every time in accordance with the external circumstances, and therefore no longer elicited separation distress. Because of his unfolding capabilities of conceptual perspective taking, he was now able to set these feelings inside a more complex differentiation of attributes between himself and his parents. Therefore, what he felt was a sense of being forced to look after himself in a social world perceived as affectively unreliable. His attitude toward his little brother not only shows clearly how the attitude toward reality was consistent with that self-image, but also evidenced an early and still rough concept of affection as protection and relief from the distress of solitude.

To what extent does the tacit knowledge of preschool years influence the lifespan development? This question resurrects the well-known debate concerning the regulating function of early experience (Hunt, 1979; Rutter, 1972, 1979).

The tendency of the classic behavioristic approach was to deny any important role to specific patterns of early experiences, while conversely, the psychoanalytic approach charged practically any early experience with a global significance, implying that during the first 5 or 6 years of life an individual's personality becomes more or less crystallized. A growing body of evidence, however, indicates that, although some early experiences may be global in nature, the vast majority of them are highly specific and related only to certain aspects of development at certain time periods. Furthermore, most early experiences, in themselves and without any relation to a specific context, would not bear any remarkable consequence unless subsequent experiences come to confirm and stabilize them (Wachs & Gruen, 1982).

In a systems/process-oriented approach, early experiences are crucial insofar as they establish children's first emotional and conceptual schemata that allow an early stable representation of self and the world. These representational patterns, in turn, become the "criterion images" against which the continuous stimulus inflow is matched and ordered. Essentially they regulate the unfolding of later lifespan developmental steps without determining them. To use a metaphor that adequately summarizes these concepts, we could say that at the end of the preschool period, a "developmental pathway" (Bowlby, 1973) emerges that by no means determines the "destination" or the "map" of the "journey" just begun, but still supplies an influential "guide" for its becoming.

CHILDHOOD

With the advent of childhood, conceptualization processes become more differentiated than the sensory–perceptual qualities indicative of the preschool years, and embrace the Piagetian stage of "concrete operations."

Children are now able to grasp a situation in an articulated way and to describe its unique elements. This undoubtedly implies a step forward toward a disengagement from the immediacy of experience—that is, decentering. Nevertheless, children's thinking is still characterized by a certain degree of object-boundness, for at this stage, verbalization cannot be detached from the designated concrete qualities of the items. At the concrete operational level, abstraction essentially involves the ability to consciously isolate one or more concrete elements in a whole, complex situation (e.g., muscular strength, number of toy soldiers, etc) and employ these elements as criteria for organizing a unity of meaning (e.g., personal worth). Concrete abstraction reaches its final equilibrium at the age of 11 years, when it is progressively replaced by formal abstraction, in which cognition becomes completely independent from the concrete situation (Strauss & Lewin, 1981).

We shall now examine how the organization of cognitive development proceeds and takes form through the phenomenal understanding of self and reality peculiar to childhood.

Parent–Child Relationship

The interdependence between complementarity and the search for autonomy becomes more complex during childhood. On one hand, concrete abstractions and a more articulated conceptual perspective taking make identification processes more complex and consolidated. On the other hand, through the formation of a social network of one's own—schoolmates, peer group, and so on—the search for autonomy acquires more definite ways of expression than the mere exploration of a physical environment and struggle for self-mastery typical of the preschool age.

In reference to identification processes, significant emotional involvement is still necessary to facilitate modeling effects, since the child's cognition is as yet very much object-bound. Unlike adolescence, at this stage, conceptual perspective taking is not developed enough for fully recognizing and differentiating one's feelings and opinions from those of significant models. The limits of concrete abstraction are therefore overcome by the vehicle of emotional arousal, which provides the child with an immediate and direct tacit understanding of the other person (Hoffman, 1975, 1978).

Therefore, the child will very probably choose as a principal model the parent with whom he/she has the more intense emotional relationship, apart from the negative or positive quality of the involvement. Because children are to a large extent active producers of their development, they may actively manipulate the level of emotional stimulation in the relationship with their parents, preferring to be beaten or punished rather than ignored. Therefore, even a negative relationship with an authoritative and punitive parent may provide an empathic arousal intense enough to foster modeling processes. It goes without saying that identification processes are carried out mainly through a tacit construction in which the child's explicit, intentional aspects play a minor role, essentially because they are not completely developed.

Because of the still-existing close complementarity of the P-C relationship, parents can considerably influence the way in which children learn to decode and recognize their own emotional experiences. Whenever the child's personal experience differs from the parents' explanation of the feelings they suppose the child is having, thoughts and emotions that have been already produced are excluded, and the parents' redefinition of them is likely to be further processed (Bowlby, 1979, 1985). We can exemplify this concept, keeping in mind how children are much more intensely and immediately attached to things than adults are (Csikszentmihalyi & Rochberg-Halton, 1981): Following a family's move to another house, a child's feelings of sadness and sense of loss over being separated from a beloved environment may be denied and redefined by the parents as happiness over the fact that, after so many sacrifices, they finally own a more comfortable home. In other words, the typical scheme is: "It's not true that you feel emotion x. You are still too young to understand it, but what you really feel is emotion y."

These situations can have considerable repercussions on developing patterns of self-perception. On the one hand, they can contribute to the exclusion of a whole range of emotional experiences from one's perceived identity, so that it will be consistent with the image that the parents seem to accept more favorably; on the other hand, they create a feeling of unreliability concerning one's ability to recognize and define properly one's own internal states.

Parents' influence is partially counterbalanced by the child's own social network of other significant relationships (teachers, peers, etc.). In fact, the progressive differentiation and articulation of the child's hierarchical range of significant models, implying an increasing emotional decentering from parents, is the most relevant aspect in the search for autonomy typical of childhood.

But, here again, the patterns of family interaction can indirectly facilitate or interfere with children's construction of their social world. The quality and consistency of *emotional aspects* of parental behavior influence the child's ability to cope with the arousal of interpersonal emotions, either magnifying or reducing possibilities of establishing significant social relations that can produce appreciable modeling effects. In addition, the quality and consistency of parents' *educational strategies* influences children's sense of competence by making them feel more or less confident in their ability to adhere to their internal standards (Crandall & Crandall, 1983). The use of affection and inductive discipline, rather than authoritarian assertions or threats of love withdrawal, fosters greater reliance on internal standards and increases the hypothesis-testing approach in reasoning (Hoffman, 1978; Leahy, 1981).

Identification Processes and the Role of Parents

Around the end of the preschool years, the child acquires a specific and quite stable gender identity (Money & Ehrhardt, 1972; Rosen & Rekers, 1980). At the same time, relations with parents also become further differentiated according to sex differences, and have distinct effects on the developing child.[3]

Identification with the parent of the same sex (or with an alternative model) is a fundamental process throughout childhood for developing the attributes of masculinity and femininity through which one's identity is immediately felt and recognized. In addition, children's self-esteem is closely associated with their relationships with the homologous parent (Crase, Foss, & Colbert, 1981; Dickstein, 1977; Dickstein & Posner, 1978).

The parent of the opposite sex, far from being less important, plays an essential role in the formation of proper interpersonal and evaluative domains inherent to one's being a male or female. In other words, as the individual approaches sexual maturation, the parent of the opposite sex can acquire the important role of "testing bench," on which the child weighs the acceptability and lovableness of his/her own gender identity. In girls, for example, the father's absence is associated with difficulties in interacting with male peers and adult men, and evidence suggests that in many cases these difficulties can be long lasting (Hetherington, 1972; Wachs & Gruen, 1982).

Obviously, the quality and consistency with which parents exhibit their sexual roles have great relevance for the development of children's reliance on their masculinity or femininity; if the parent's behavior is rigid, ambiguous, or unpredictable, the entire process is slower and more uncertain, with the possible emergence of an equivocal sense of lovableness and a precarious self-esteem.

The Emergence of Stable Boundaries of the Self

As we have seen, at the end of preschool years, the first stable ensemble of nuclear scenes begins to differentiate itself into clusters of emotional schemata ordered in a recursive loop that oscillate between opponent boundaries of meaning. We can now proceed to analyze how, during childhood and through the emerging of new cognitive abilities, this basic recursive loop becomes increasingly differentiated and articulated.

For the sake of a more fluent discussion, I shall first discuss in general terms the interplay between emotional differentiation and cognitive growth. Next, I will describe the articulated and complex regulation between opponent boundaries of the self that emerges from this interplay. This subdivision is of course only adopted to simplify the exposition, since in reality we are dealing with a dynamic process characterized by the embeddedness of its levels of analyses.

Emotional Differentiation and Cognitive Growth

The interplay between emotional and cognitive development can be regarded as a self-enhancing process in which patterns of experience are scaffolded through the existing tacit boundaries of meaning. These "boundaries" function as deep ordering rules that structure the invariant aspects of a person's mental processing and maximize coherence and internal consistency by extracting only specific patterns of regularity and excluding all others.

Emotional differentiation and further articulation of nuclear scenes can, therefore, be viewed as a progressive matching process between preformed emotional schemata and ongoing feelings. The *search for coherence*, guided by the assimilation of actual feelings within the existing ensemble of emotional schemata, regulates and provides continuity to the forward-in-time motion of the entire process. When certain feelings cannot be assimilated, the perception of this discrepancy acts as the main elicitor for differentiating new emotional domains along the continuum between boundaries of meaning. These patterns of emotional schemata, in turn, influence available cognitive abilities to structure an ordered set of beliefs and thoughts—procedures that govern, control, and further articulate the patterns themselves, making their tacit content more explicit.

The global nature of this process cannot be encompassed by traditional developmental approaches that merely focus on limited aspects of cognitive functioning. More integrative conceptual devices, capable of assembling single cognitive abilities into ordered wholes and explaining the logic and coherence of children's behavior, are needed. Presently, the notion of "script" seems to offer promise as such an integrative device (Abelson, 1981; Schank & Abelson, 1977).

A script is essentially a bundle of expectations that directs cognitive processing toward an appropriate comprehension of specific situations through the simultaneous activation of a set of conceived events, any of which may become involved in a particular inference (Abelson, 1981, p. 717). Whenever a magnified scene elicits the generation of a script, the activation of both the ensemble of emotional schemata and the set of conceptual rules for decoding and controlling them organizes the whole interaction of the individual with the relevant situation (Tomkins, 1978). The case of Eric who, at 5 years of age, reacted to a situation that he perceived as desertion by protecting his smaller brother, is a typical instance of how a script governs a nuclear scene, while at the same time it allows one to understand his/her emotions and to plan actions consistently with that understanding. It should be specified that a script not only has a decoding and controlling function but, more important, it regulates the intensity and quality of underlying emotional schemata by making them more explicit, and thus influences to a large extent both the form they assume and their further articulation.

In conclusion, the interplay between emotional and cognitive development in childhood can be depicted as a progressive differentiation of emotional domains along the self-recursive loop, paralleled by an interdependent set of organized cognitive structures (scripts) that explicates the ongoing implicit ordering into beliefs, automatic habits, and interpersonal attitudes.

The Oscillative Regulation between Boundaries of the Self

Due to the progressive differentiation of the child's self-recursive loop, opponent process regulation becomes increasingly articulated and resilient, allowing for smooth, "round-trip" oscillations between boundaries of meaning. In contrast to the initial perceptions that prompted the original recursive loop, this permits a flexible understanding of a variety of complex situations.

Returning to the example of an early recursive loop centered on helplessness and anger, rapid oscillations between the two opponent boundaries are practically the rule in preschool years. It is as though reality can only be understood through recurring and alternating desertions and reactions to desertions. Later in childhood, helplessness and anger become mingled together through an articulated range of emotions—sadness, nostalgia, indifference, curiosity, excitement, and so on—so that the child is able to moderate painful emotional extremes by actively seeking these intermediate states via the elaboration of specific scripts; for example, a passive, sad sense of self explicated through an appeasing interpersonal attitude enables the child to avoid or check immoderate emotionality connected to both rejection and his/her reactions to rejections.

The attempt to integrate two different perceived senses of self through the tendency toward intermediate states represents the ongoing dynamic equilibrium resulting from the mutual integration of opponent boundaries of meaning that constrain one another. During childhood, therefore, the regulating mechanisms that mold an adaptive coalition of decentralized control processes become more clear-cut.

Selfhood processes differentiate themselves as a coalition of mutually interacting structures embedded within a context of interdependent boundary constraints, with no single locus in ultimate control (Mahoney, in press; Weimer, 1983). At the developmental level, coalitional control parallels very well Waddington's (1957, 1977) idea of "epigenesis" at the evolutionary level; at any moment, the ongoing actual self expresses the dynamic, developmental pathway resulting from the integration of simultaneous but different pressures. Paraphrasing Waddington's epigenetic landscape, co-alitional control enables the developing self to right itself after a perturbation and return to its former track.

At present, the regulative mechanisms underlying the structuring of specific patterns of coalitional control are scarcely investigated and poorly understood. However, a promising attempt in that direction is offered by the information-processing model of defense mechanisms proposed by Bowlby (1980a), whose ideas I draw upon.

1. The ongoing developmental pathway expressed by actual patterns of coalitional control is buffered against specific perturbation by selectively excluding sensory inflow coming from critical domains.

The excluding capacity obviously depends on the degree of available cognitive abilities. In young children, excluding procedures are mainly direct, and incoming inflow is, in a way, not consciously registered. Therefore, they seem to exclude inflow more readily than older children. However, young children's immediacy limits the flexibility of their adaptation and makes them more vulnerable to complex, ambiguous situations, whereas older children can use excluding procedures that are more indirect and cognitively mediated. For example, they are able to change the sensory inflow or assimilate it into an inadequate conceptual frame. This makes them more resilient and protected in assimilating painful perturbations.

Whenever a child is faced with intense and not easily avoidable perturbations, exclusion often reaches dramatic levels of intensity, bringing about what Bowlby calls the "cognitive disconnection" of a response from the interpersonal situation that elicited it. When the disconnection is complete, the response appears completely unintelligible in terms of one's reactions and can be better explained by attributing it to external causes like somatic or psychological complaints.

Throughout development, therefore, the selective exclusion of inflow deeply influences the elaboration of a very personal range of perceivable emotions, the only ones youngsters can recognize as their own.

2. Any perturbation usually exerts pressures for shifting the actual, ongoing self toward one of its boundaries—for example, to react to threats of desertion or love withdrawal with outbursts of anger. Needless to say, if the child succeeds in systematically

excluding critical inflow, anger and scripts related to it are prevented from being activated.

However, in cases in which exclusion is incomplete, the pressures for such a shift can be circumvented through the activation of other feelings, thoughts, and behaviors that increase a child's control by changing his/her focus of attention. Children may busy themselves with some form of activity that diverts them from further processing the information that is being excluded. These activities that sometimes take the form of clear-cut symptoms—psychosomatic disturbances, rituals, phobias, overeating, etc.—have been incisively called "diversionary activities" by Bowlby:

> They give the impression, on the one hand, of being carried out under pressure and of absorbing an undue proportion of a person's attention, time and energy, perhaps in the form of overwork, and, on the other, of being undertaken by him in some way at the expense of his giving his attention, time and energy to something else. They seem thus to be not merely alternatives but also to be playing a diversionary role; and this is probably what they do. (1980a, p. 66)

Thus, throughout development, deactivation of opponent systems and diversionary activity play a crucial role in the elaboration of a repertoire of automatic cognitive–emotional reactions that help to immobilize the subject in the face of an impending challenge to his/her sense of identity.

Selfhood Processes in Childhood

The first part of childhood is characterized by the differentiation of a rather stable ongoing self out of the interplay of cognitive–emotional processes. However, conceptual perspective taking is linked to concrete abstractions, and children are still bound, to some extent, to ongoing emotional attachments in order to support their sense of self (Montemayor & Eisen, 1977). This condition, which is apt to become more pronounced in cases of intrusive, ambiguous, or repressive attachments, can not only limit the child's cognitive resilience, but, in some circumstances, it may hinder his/her growing sense of independency and autonomy.

Brenda, age 40, a severely obese housewife, had grown up in close contact with her mother, whose attitude toward her was constantly ambiguous; she expected from Brenda a mature, self-controlling behavior, but at the same time she treated her like a fickle infant, incapable of checking herself. The mother's attitude was also rather intruding and overcontrolling, she always defined Brenda's emotions in advance, and suggested how to control them.

This enmeshed pattern of attachment contributed to the development of Brenda's self-boundaries, which loosely wavered between the opponent polarities of being "externally bound" (perceived as utter unreliability and uncompetence) and trying to be "internally bound" (which she perceived as dreadfully blurred). As often happens in these cases (see Chapter 9), Brenda succeeded in finding a steady and dynamic adaptative equilibrium. Her actual self was differentiated by maintaining her mother as the essential point of reference, but at the same time controlling *her own* emotional expression and displaying self-sufficient attitudes, thus recovering a more defined sense of demarcation from her mother.

At age 7, Brenda underwent surgery in order to have her tonsils removed. When Brenda woke up from the anesthesia following the operation, she saw her mother smiling and saying that everything was all right and that she needn't worry, since her mouth and throat had simply been "photographed." The child felt perfectly calm and felt *no* pain whatsoever in her throat. But, soon after, her mother gravely told her it had all been a joke, and that since the operation had taken more time than was expected, she should probably feel a little fatigued. *Suddenly* Brenda felt acute pains in her throat, and proceeded to cry uncontrollably—something she rarely did.

During this sudden change in the situation, Brenda probably experienced exactly the kind of emotional dependency and motherbound attitude that she carefully tried to exclude from her mental processing. It is interesting to note that this event apparently had no remarkable consequence on Brenda's behavior.

This gap between a direct and immediate emotional experience and its conscious explicit restructuring is characteristic of the first phase of childhood. While children elaborate rules, beliefs, and opinions about themselves and the people that surround them, the cognitive structuring of these rules cannot go beyond the specific context in which they originated. Studies on metacognitive development clearly support the hypothesis that children (unlike early adolescents and youths) do not monitor their memory and communication or their perceptions and appraisals (Flavell, 1977, 1978, 1979).

These conditions undoubtedly facilitate a direct exclusion of significant input; however, this does not mean that experiences of this nature have no repercussions at the tacit organizing level. When already-formed emotional schemata are excluded from subsequent processing, their later conceptualization becomes impossible; that is, they cannot be transformed into objects of thought. Nevertheless, they are very likely to influence emotional differentiation, contributing to the exclusion of definite feelings from one's conscious emotional range, and to the establishment of a sense of unreliability in one's own emotional and intellectual abilities, as well as a basic mistrust in other people's intentions. It should be emphasized that Brenda related this episode during therapy to demonstrate the affection she and her mother had for each other, and she therefore gave it a positive, rather than a negative, connotation. She could not, however, explain the strange sense of awkwardness she felt every time she remembered the event.

Cognitive abilities become disengaged from concrete abstractions only at the upper elementary age (9–11 years), when the Piagetian stage of preformal operations shifts conceptual perspective taking to a more abstract level. The consequences of such a shift are remarkable. For example, while younger children tend to attribute to others characteristics that belong to themselves, by now a sense of others as having their own personal identities and inner states begins to emerge. The focus on the immediate situation, therefore, is gradually reduced and the older child is able to respond not only to others' specific and transitory situations, but also to what he/she imagines to be their large pattern of life experiences.

This, of course, also implies a change in the sense of self. The attainment of higher semantic levels of information processing allows for the emergence of a sense of past and future, since abstract conceptualization most likely makes it possible to assign a temporal and historical dimension to ongoing data. Consequently, while the sense of temporal becoming remains hazy up until 9 years of age, the older child develops the capacity to integrate his/her own discrete inner experiences with respect to the passage of time. As a result, a sense of self emerges as having different feelings and thoughts in different situations but being the same, continuous person with his/her own past, present, and anticipated future (Hoffman, 1975).

At the age of 10, Brenda had an unpleasant accident one evening at dinner. She had taken too large a mouthful of food, and it went the wrong way, causing her to have a protracted dyspnea crisis. Brenda remembered clearly that she had not felt too scared about the event itself, since she had seen it happen to other people without serious consequences. What did shock Brenda was the terrified expression on her mother's face (she was usually a very controlled person) while she made senseless efforts to make the daughter expel the mouthful. That was when Brenda felt she was going through something extremely serious, perhaps irreparable. Obviously, shortly after the incident was over, with no further consequence, dinner proceeded as usual. Brenda, however, soon developed a strong anorexic reaction that lasted about one year and kept her away from school for long periods. She ate little food, had bizarre tastes, and would eat only by herself, in the kitchen, and outside of mealtimes. During therapy, Brenda reported the episode as a curious anecdote that she could only explain by saying: "Apparently, I had become afraid of eating."

As we can see, although Brenda had found herself in a situation similar to the one that followed the tonsillectomy, she reacted in a completely different way; experiencing again an emotional mother-bound attitude, she magnified immediately her opponent regulation processes. Through the diversionary activity of anorexic behavior, Brenda was first able to increase and later to recover the usual control over herself.

The most relevant aspect in late childhood is, therefore, the emergence of a cognitive sense of others as distinct from the acting self, who, in turn, is more and more able to impose his/her own ordering processes upon reality. This aspect may be expected to expand considerably through adolescence and youth.

ADOLESCENCE AND YOUTH

The emergence of logical, abstract thought (Piagetian stage of "formal operations") appears to be of utmost importance to the marked differentiation and integration of selfhood processes occurring during adolescence and youth. To rid thought of the *immediacy* of the situation is to elaborate a superordinate conceptual coding that becomes the essential framework for creating hypotheses and making inferences (Bernstein, 1980; Strauss & Lewin, 1981).

Hence, the most important property of logical/deductive thinking concerns the relationship between *what is real* and *what is possible*: Perceived reality comes to be conceived of as a particular subset within the totality of events and things. This implies a true "widening of the world," as adolescents can now grasp the existence of aspects of reality that are different from those they personally experience, inferring them by means of hypotheses and causal theories. The subordination of the real world to the possible world, while orienting the attention toward problems that go beyond the phenomenal experience, also modifies the concept of time, and especially of the future, which now loses the vagueness and indefiniteness of childhood.

The discussion of this remarkable personal rearrangement proceeds along the same levels of analysis that have been taken into consideration for previous stages.

Parent–Adolescent Relationship

Through adolescence and youth, the patterns of family interaction are subject to significant changes, that further modify the interplay between complementarity and the search for autonomy in parent–adolescent (P-A) relations (Steinberg, 1981; Steinberg & Hill, 1978).

Identification Processes

The new cognitive abilities make identification processes somewhat different from what they were in preschool years and childhood.

Because of a less emotion-bound attitude in interpersonal relationships, the adolescent's struggle to acquire a satisfactory adult identity directs identification processes toward the internalization of a model's life values and existential–philosophical axioms. Logical/deductive processing permits an attunement to even more abstract units of knowledge, most of which are assimilated mainly in a tacit way. Tacitly acquired knowledge units function as reference criteria in the matching processes through which a greater integration between the individual and his/her perceived future is carried out, and thus play a major role in the construction of the person's life programming.

Therefore, regardless of the emotional quality of ongoing attachments, adolescent identification processes produce a tacit coding of reality out of the mother's or father's perceived values; but these are not realized until later, when as adults, they face events and situations determined by that coding. Here again, though, parental influence is fairly well counterbalanced by other significant social relationships. In fact, thanks to the ability to grasp the essence of a given situation apart from its immediate aspects, such relationships now allow adolescents to find alternative sentimental, ideological, and social commitments to those embodied by their parents.

It is also well known that in adolescence and youth the individual experiences a more or less complete cognitive and emotional separation from his/her parents; although in most cases, this does not necessarily imply a true physical separation. It should not be assumed, however, that separation progressively reduces identification processes. On the contrary, evidence supports the notion that separation works as a primary motivation for identification (Bloom, 1980). Since internalization increases in response to any kind of separation or loss (Bowlby, 1980a; Parkes, 1972), during and after separation from parents, modeling processes are more or less tacitly enhanced. This enables the adolescent to acquire a more organized patterning of parental values. As Levinson (1970) incisively argued, it is as though the primary value of a relationship were, in a way, created *after it ends*—yet another example, we may assume, of opponent regulation processes. Thus, despite their opposite tendencies, identification and separation are not in themselves antagonistic in the sense that if one is stronger, one would expect the other to be weaker. On the contrary, they are *interdependent*; and an adequate identification is a crucial variable in fostering a proper search for autonomy, since it is identification itself that maintains the feeling of one's continuity during and after the whole separation process.

The Search for Autonomy

As adolescents progress in their development, they start to take a completely different view of their parents. In childhood, and even more in preschool years, parents appear to hold unquestionable truths and values; whereas now, due to the relativism of adolescent thought, they are perceived more or less as ordinary people possessing the usual uncertainties, problems, and idiosyncrasies. They are considered less essential in supporting and confirming one's sense of identity; their position as primary attachment figures decreases; and this, in turn, starts the process of cognitive–emotional separation.

The P-A separation, although a normal process at this stage of development, seems to follow a step-by-step, oscillative pattern similar to any separation or loss process (Bowlby, 1973, 1980a; Parkes, 1972). In other words, through a sequence of cognitive transformations (e.g., decentration, enhancing of internalization, and their final balancing) intermeshed with corresponding emotions (e.g., anger, guilt, and autonomy), adolescents experience a growing number of interruptions of the ongoing attachment to their parents, eventually reaching an adult identity matched by a new attitude toward others.

As Bloom (1980) remarked, the P-A separation is the first separation experience that the person undertakes with personal and cultural awareness and under the influence of personal development; and therefore, it can be considered as the prototypic separation in life. That is, it may function as a reference criterion in the making and matching processes for understanding and facing subsequent separations and losses of adult life, such as the end of a significant relationship or the death of a loved one.

As attachment to parents becomes less central, affective sexual relationships rise in importance, since adolescents seek in them the support and confirmation of their sense of identity that they previously sought from parental attachments. Therefore, an adaptive love life in youth is the coherent consequence of an adequate and well-balanced development of both identification and separation, and represents the most direct expression of the competence and autonomy reached by the developing individual. As clinical experience confirms, difficulties in maintaining or establishing emotional involvements with others—usually a consequence of abnormal patterns of family attachment and corresponding distorted identification processes—indicate an uncertain sense of competence and autonomy and a precarious commitment toward life (Biller, 1974; Hetherington, 1972; Hetherington & Parke, 1979; Wachs & Gruen, 1982).[4]

The Reorganization of Self-Boundaries

In reaching adolescence, an individual's selfhood processes are already endowed with a structured tendency toward the moment-to-moment attainment of a rather stable oscillative equilibrium between boundaries of personal meaning, reflecting the differentiation of a repertoire of automatic cognitive–emotional reactions that buffer ongoing perturbations.

The adolescent "revolution" is represented by *qualitative* transformations of the individual self-system. Various ensembles of emotional schemata and the scripts related to them are continually rehearsed, re-elaborated, and matched with the novel experiences stemming from logical/deductive thinking, sexual maturation, and autonomy (separation from parents). Of course, this does not mean that we should underestimate the creation of new and original knowledge units, since any emergent level of selfhood processes contains novelties that cannot be reduced to the previous level, even though the latter held them in its range of developmental possibilities. Emphasis is given to the qualitative aspect only because it seems to be a distinctive feature of adolescence and youth; no other phase of the whole lifespan—except perhaps the occurrence of a true "personal revolution" (Mahoney, 1980)—undergoes such qualitative and simultaneous transformations on several levels as does this period.

Following the same procedure as in previous analyses, we can now discuss how logical/deductive processing capabilities first influence the interplay between emotional and cognitive development, and later the reorganization of the coalitional control of self-structures out of this interplay.

Emotional–Cognitive Interplay

The co-assembly of emotional schemata and related scripts provides the developing child with an apperceptive scaffolding that constrains immediate experience and makes it understandable. Because abstract thought carries attention beyond immediacy, it is no longer sufficient to grasp the sense of experience. It is the meaning of life itself that now must be understood—that is, *what reality can be and how we are related to it.*

Such an epistemological shift entails the elaboration of metaphysical assumptions about reality. Following from Broughton's (1981) insightful assertion that knowledge must always be of some reality, it could similarly be argued that any epistemology presupposes a metaphysics. Thus, on the one hand, the abstracting process is directed to specific *rules* (e.g., scripts) for dealing with emotional experiences that are converted into *axioms* ordered in a coherent framework that explain how reality can produce those particular experiences. On the other hand, this emerging conception of reality is projected in a now well-developed sense of time that provides a predictability over the future comparable to very complex scientific theories.

In fact, this abstracting ability is matched by the differentiation of a reflexive dimension of consciousness, that is, a rather stable conscious monitoring of oneself (self-awareness). The awakening of self-awareness, in turn, entails the separation of present into future, present, and past, allowing for the historical and temporal structuring of ongoing experience (Watanabe, 1972). In other words, as generally transpires in the development of complex systems, a "symmetry-breaking" process (Jantsch, 1980; Prigogine, 1973) has occurred—that is, a break of the static symmetry between past and future (typical until late childhood), and the projection of the emergent, irreversible directionality of time into cognitive processes. This gives rise to a personal, subjective transformation of time, parallel and interwoven with the objective temporal realm. Needless to say, a symmetry-breaking process unfolds a new space–time dimension that affects the reorganization of selfhood processes and makes available new knowledge abilities and experience domains.

The integrative notion of "metascript" (Schank & Abelson, 1977) represents a useful conceptual tool for understanding the effect of abstract processing on the co-assembly of emotional schemata and related scripts. According to Abelson (1981), the defining feature of a "metascript" is that, due to further processing, many of its emotional schemata and rules are specified at a higher level of abstraction than are those of scripts. For example, an adolescent girl's scripts governing the emotional schemata elicited by love withdrawal by a beloved father may be abstracted into a *metascript* consisting of various superordinate principles pertaining to mate selection and strategies for controlling affective relations. This metatascript would help her manage the emotions aroused by the experience of being abandoned, which, in turn, has resulted in her believing is more than likely to occur in such relationships.

It is emotional experience that turns scripts into generalized metascripts that, in turn, can modify the intensity and quality of emotional schemata. Affect, besides being the only immediate and relevant self-referent information available, is inherently consistent over time. Therefore, it is hardly surprising, that both scripts and metascripts are organized around basic ensembles of emotional schemata (nuclear scenes) and their ever growing differentiation (Izard, 1980; Izard & Buechler, 1980, 1983; Tomkins, 1978).

The Rearrangement of Adolescent Self

As we have mentioned, reorganization concerns not so much the *contents* of structured boundaries of meaning, as the *way* in which their reordering, according to emerging higher semantic dimensions, affects the individual's self and world perception.

The new epistemological relationship between the knower and reality is primarily reflected by two simultaneous, interdependent and complementary processes: (1) *decentering from the world* and (2) *recentering on the self* (Chandler, 1975; Turner, 1973).

1. The discovery of a multiplicity of possible viewpoints behind the apparent oneness of the phenomenological world, necessarily implies a more relativistic view of reality. This requires a turning away from the immediacy of emotional involvement with people and events, except for specific domains of experience tied to peer groups and affective partners. It is a common observation that the precariousness or unreliability of these domains is responsible for the dreariest feelings of loneliness and despair in teenagers.

In a way, reality appears more "real" at the cost of being depersonalized, and this decentered attitude toward reality carries as a consequence a new perception of the individual's oneness and uniqueness that Chandler (1975) very appropriately called "sense of epistemological loneliness."

2. In order to govern the emergent sense of epistemological loneliness, adolescents have to put their sense of self and life at the center of all their moment-to-moment personal experiencing. That is, while acknowledging the plurality of alternative perspectives, the subject must commit him/herself to some perspective and meaning felt as uniquely personal. Thus, the commitment to oneself is paralleled by the life programming of one's perceived future—an essential aspect of metascripts processing—that allows the subject to resume an ongoing involvement with the same reality. In addition to this sense of epistemological loneliness, the oscillation between decentering and recentering gives rise to another range

of emerging, challenging feelings that increase pressures toward a steady commitment to oneself.

While the deep oscillation between self-boundaries, on one side, and the tendency toward intermediate states, on the other, do not reach the sphere of personal awareness until childhood, the advent of adolescence is accompanied by the emergence of a felt dichotomy between a perceived "apparent self" (the way we behave in specific situations) and a perceived "real self" (the way we feel no matter what the situation may be) (Broughton, 1981). The unveiling of this split awareness—an authentically new dimension whose continuous equilibration will become one of the main themes of later adult life—is a sign of the dawning consciousness of the opponent regulation between decentering and recentering. In effect, we may assume that the apparent self is the action of perceiving the self through its concrete, moment-to-moment instantiations (decentering), while the real self is the perception of oneself as being immediately and directly affected by one's inner boundaries, regardless of its subsequent instantiations (recentering).

Therefore, adolescence and youth may be regarded as a search for *dynamic balance*—the first stable integration between different senses of self, representing the progression of an individual's coalitional control toward higher levels of abstraction and reflexive consciousness. This integration occurs simultaneously in the present and in the anticipated future, so that the different senses of self are recognized, transversally, as belonging to the same person and are connected in an overall relationship that has as its *longitudinal expression* the real self (life programming), and as its concrete, *immediate expression* the apparent self. The commitment to oneself, as the emergent result of the balancing between the tendency to decenter from the world and the tendency to recenter on the self, represents a crucial lifespan integration, since it corresponds to the initial programming of one's life theme.

Returning to the metaphor of an individual lifespan being like a journey, it could be said that while the early construction of a developmental pathway (around the end of preschool years) only suggested a preferable directionality for the trip, with no other specifications, with adolescence, *begins a commitment* to a map of possible goals and probable ways and means of reaching them is begun. The quality of the possible life themes and the degree of clearness with which they can be perceived depend of course on the abstracting ability at the time of adolescent reorganization.

In the lives of remarkable men, adolescence and early youth can, in most cases, be recognized as milestones for their focusing on what will later be the central theme of their lives. Einstein, for example, was 16 years old when, watching the sunlight mirrored by the surface of a lake, he was suddenly struck by the amazing insight that in order to grasp the still unknown aspects of the universe, one should imagine traveling at the speed of light (Clark, 1971). Popper, at 17 years of age, apparently as a reaction to his first social and political disappointments, had already begun to clearly outline his theme on the falsifiability of scientific theories, which later became a fundamental point of reference for epistemologists (Popper, 1974).

Even in more ordinary people, the attained level of abstraction can be observed to influence, though to a less striking degree, the quality and genuineness of adolescence's commitment. Evidence taken from the analysis of life histories (Csikszentmihalyi & Beattie, 1979) shows that a main dimension of an individual lifespan is the extent to which, during adolescence, the emergence of a new appraisal of self and world is actively "discovered" (i.e., experienced as volitionally imposing one's view upon reality) as opposed to passively "accepted" (i.e., experienced as adapting oneself to an externally defined view of the world). In the first instance—relating as a rule to people who, regardless of their unhappy childhood, were successful in life—a greater abstraction ability allowed the person to develop on his/her own the themes around which commitment could be built; whereas, in the second case, available cognitive abilities seemed to allow only an acceptance of ready-made themes supplied by the familial environment.

Paraphrasing a famous psychoanalytic tenet in light of the present perspective, it could be stated that the crux of a lifespan is to be found not so much in the first 5 years of life, as more probably in how the adolescent integration is accomplished and in the quality and genuineness of its consequent commitment. Being a complex rebalancing operation between opponent aspects of selfhood processes, this integration is seldom painless and in some cases produces maladaptive, precarious self-integrations. Apart from cases of "difficult" adolescences that can, sometimes, be a prelude to original, creative personalities in adult life, clinical experience has shown that adolescence is one of the "high-risk" life periods for the onset of clear-cut clinical syndromes.

Finally, the adolescent achievement of repersonalizing reality, once it becomes marked by relativity, presumably can be considered as the first, prototypical integration in an individual's lifespan of a "physiological" deep change—that is, it may work in a person's life as a reference criterion against which are matched subsequent challenges for deep changes or personal revolutions.

Selfhood Processes in Adolescence and Youth

Adolescence represents a crucial developmental step, because depending on how its maturational transformations are integrated, individuals will either have fewer or greater possibilities of developing a genuine commitment to themselves, and this, in turn, will influence most of their future lifespan.

In this concluding section of this chapter, the significance of this developmental period will be exemplified primarily through the use of clinical vignettes, since they provide substance to some general considerations about development. These vignettes provide a means for summarizing the central propositions up to this point and for highlighting some of the patterns and processes that facilitate the emergence of adult cognitive dysfunctions, discussed more extensively in Part 3. Because separation and autonomy from parents, better than any other process, can be taken as a phenomenal indicant of the course and quality of underlying adolescent integrative processes, cases reported here will be considered mainly from this point of view. Although the ways of interfering with the separation process are many and can vary from case to case, their basic mechanism is roughly the same. Abnormal patterns of attachment interfere with identification processes by bringing about the structuring of distorted self-conceptions, through which a sufficient degree of inner coherence is ensured only by means of an increased exclusion of emotions and experiences. This exclusion keeps identification processes at an immediate and object-bound level resembling that of childhood. Thus, one's attitude toward reality becomes a critical factor, especially at the time when the need for autonomy and independence is increasing.

Derek, a 38-year-old obsessive lawyer, had a very peculiar family pattern of attachment. His father, who was also a lawyer, had no part whatever in the family life; Derek's mother was his second wife, and he put her in charge of the entire household, including two small children from the previous marriage. The mother, Derek's true attachment figure, was a fervent Catholic and a morally rigid person. Ever since Derek was born, she was firmly resolved, for the sake of justice toward the other two children, not to feel the slightest emotion in favor of her own child. Her decision "not to feel" emotions—which by their nature are inescapable and unavoidable—brought paradoxical consequences. Since she *did* feel a preference for Derek (and her decision not to feel it was, indeed, a sign of it), she forced herself to show a marked preference for her stepchildren, punishing Derek each time with either physical punishments or love withdrawals, and making him appear in any circumstance as the "black sheep."

On the other hand, Derek knew that he was his mother's favorite if for no other reason than because she, usually so self-controlled and uneffusive, seemed much more involved with him than with any other member of the family. For example, after she had beaten him for minor matters, she would suddenly burst into tears and hug and kiss him warmly.

The antithetic aspects of his mother's attachment—love at the tacit level and rejection at the explicit one—puzzled Derek during early childhood when his available cognitive abilities were limited. Only with the emergence in late childhood of preformal operations did Derek, who knew about the family situation, sense that the problem had a moral and religious origin. He then suddenly became meditative, controlled, and religious in order to legitimize his relationship with his mother within a common moral context. He had, in a way, decided to protect his mother from his emotional involvement, which, with the concrete self-referent logic of his age, he perceived as the source of all their problems.

During youth, Derek was strongly attached to girls, especially older ones, but he soon had difficulties in establishing any defined emotional commitment. As soon as each relationship started, he would become strongly doubtful about his involvement, apparently because of the girl's older age—although this was actually a necessary requirement for his being interested in her. He imagined vividly how, with the passing of time, the difference in their age would become more and more evident and how, in the end, he would be attracted to other women and abandon her. This induced him in long, fruitless ruminations that he then disclosed to his partner. By repeatedly describing his ruminations, he would continually "test" the relationship, until it would finally end—usually at the initiation of the women.

Derek's case warrants a few general comments. First, it represents a good example of the shift in knowledge level that takes place during the adolescent reorganization process. While in infancy and childhood Derek had built a sense of his oneness, essentially through the attachment to his mother, the subsequent decentering and recentering of adolescence turned the same sense of oneness into a general way of coding reality that he, as actor, had now to impose on the world. Owing to the "cognitive revolution" of this period, Derek's nuclear scripts—that is, specific concrete rules to protect his mother from his emotional involvement—were turned into more abstract metascripts—that is, more abstract rules to protect women from his possible affective inconstancy.

Finally, as we can see, the process of emotional separation from parents was not complete, limiting Derek's capacity of affective commitment and, therefore, his autonomy. In his attitude toward himself and reality, Derek mainly transposed to a more abstract level the troubled relationship with his mother, as if this were still the actual ongoing involvement. To paraphrase metaphorically, it is as if, in a play of mirrors, Derek simply redirected toward reality the image of his relationship with his mother, which, in turn, reflected back a concept of the world.

Shirley, a 36-year-old agoraphobic physician, grew up in a family in which the father, himself a doctor, was the dominating figure, while the mother had always been secondary. Shirley was her father's favorite and he personally took care of her upbringing. Besides having strict rules about school accomplishments, he especially insisted on many meticulous habits that he believed would avoid diseases or accidents that seemed to him to pose a constant threat in any situation. The father himself, as sometimes happens to physicians, was a hypochondriac and suffered from several neurovegetative disorders that "forced him" to lead a rigorously methodical life. When Shirley was a teenager, her father's moralistic control immediately took over her social life. He described emotional and sexual aspects of relationships with boys as sources of possible physical and psychological breakdowns and, little by little, forced her to live in an almost monastic way. Shirley accepted this without rebelling because she felt satisfied with the exclusive, preferential affection that her father, her primary attachment figure, gave her.

When she was 15 years old, her father suddenly died of a heart attack, and Shirley, who always controlled her emotions, was apparently restrained on that occasion. When, as an adult, she talked about it in therapy, she remembered that she had felt a sense of danger, as though she were without protection and abandoned to herself, without her father's control. Because her mother had never had any influence or control over her, she left Shirley free to do what she wanted, including staying out at night. However, little by little, Shirley found that she could give herself the same control that her father expected, and, at the same time, that this was the best way to reduce the sense of his loss. She returned to her orderly, secluded life and everything went well until at age 17, she started dating a boy in her class and began to feel her first sexual arousals. In a short time she started to have panic attacks in the classroom, in school, and later in social occasions with people her age, to the point that she felt relatively calm only at home.

The analysis of Derek's case seems quite applicable to Shirley's; here, in fact, the interference in the separation process seems even more evident. Besides demonstrating how a completely different pattern of attachment may interfere with the separation process, Shirley's example was specifically chosen to show how an abrupt separation can intensify identification and stabilize it. The influence of an identification model, even in the absence of an ongoing involvement, may clearly reach beyond the maturational stages and have pervasive effects during the whole individual lifespan. This provides all the more reason to place special emphasis on the reconstruction of family attachment styles in the understanding of adult existential and clinical problems.

In other situations, autonomy from parents seems to be impaired in a more indirect way by abnormal patterns of attachment. In early development, rather than limiting exploration, they interfere with the structuring of coherent patterns for self-perception and self-evaluation; and during adolescence, they hinder the attainment of an integrated perception of one's identity. In many such circumstances it is possible to detect, even in the earliest phases of childhood, an effort on the part of the child to actively differentiate him/herself from the problematic parent. Therefore, reduced autonomy and self-competence seem to be a by-product, rather than a direct result, of attachment.

Brenda (see pp. 60, 62), for the entire course of her adolescence, succeeded in going through a process of differentiation from her mother and was finally able to impose upon herself an alternative way of considering femininity. While her mother was an idealistic woman who kept conceiving grandiose dreams of independence and personal realization, Brenda won her mother's esteem for being stern, controlled in her emotions, down-to-earth, and socially committed in a group of friends. In this way she had become the wise one in the family, and her mother often came to her for advice. Brenda was now able to master her childhood tendencies of avoiding uncontrollable emotions and withdrawing from those situations in which she either felt bound to an external definition of herself or extreme self-reliance (fearing her incompetence would show). The relationship with her mother had reached a satisfying equilibrium; while, on one hand, she received a distinct sense of her own identity from the continuous comparison with her mother, on the other hand, the diversity from her mother guaranteed a sense of independence and autonomy.

When Brenda was around 18 years old and had her first boyfriend, problems came both from the mother, disappointed in her choice and reacting with detachment and love withdrawal, and from the boyfriend, who demanded from Brenda a greater involvement. Brenda soon found herself in a state of almost complete uncertainty; she was not able to understand whether she was more interested in pursuing the relationship with her boyfriend or in maintaining her mother's good opinion of her. It was during this time that she had her first sexual experience, and she had had a similar ambiguous attitude toward it; that is, she wasn't sure whether she was following her curiosity or simply was afraid of disappointing the boyfriend. That night, while she was in her room thinking about what had happened, her mother called for her dinner. Going into the dining room Brenda caught a glimpse of her image in a mirror, and with a sense of being unable to recognize herself, perhaps forever, she panicked. A painfully sharp sensation caused her to faint for a few seconds, and the family had to call a doctor.

Brenda at once erased any recollection of these events (she recalled the episode many years later in therapy) and after a time acted in such a way that her relationship with her boyfriend came to an end. She subsequently returned to a very orderly life, but some time later started to feel, more and more often, an anxiety-eliciting inner sense of emptiness that could best be controlled by compulsive overeating.

I preferred to leave Brenda's case as the concluding one because it suggests a general consideration that is essential to grasping the developmental dynamics of selfhood processes. Specifically, our perceived identity (which for us corresponds to the sense of reality itself) finds in the presence of others a necessary foundation for its existence, and at the same time, in the differentiation from others, discovers the equally necessary foundation for its experiencing. There, in the dynamic point of intersection of the opponent regulation between an *outward tendency* to perceive the wholes of which we are a part, and an *inward tendency* to perceive the parts that make us a whole (Sameroff, 1982) we can trace the sense of our identity and uniqueness.

NOTES

1. It is well known that most sensorial–associationistic theories of mind embrace a reductionistic approach to thought, regarding it as a mere internalization of language and, therefore, just a by-product of it. This perspective, however, seems to be unquestionably disproved by the evidence that language is not an initiating cause of thought during the earliest phases of development.

Thus, from an evolutionary–epistemologic viewpoint, then, a different (and, in a way, totally opposite) hypothesis seems legitimate; namely, that when thought reaches a certain degree of evolutionary complexity in its abstracting abilities, there emerges the "epistemological" need of a new device, such as language, that allows, through a code of symbols, the articulation and conversion of abstractions into manipulatable "concretes," that is, into concepts and representations.

2. Unlike older hypotheses that considered earliest attachment to be mediated by a "dependence need" secondary to the primary hunger drive, the "contact" with a living caregiver is the fundamental mediator, as Harlow (1958) undisputably demonstrated. In accordance with the present perspective, it can be added that the *essence* of living contact facilitates the infant's molding of its basic feelings into corresponding emotional schemata by connecting them with parallel physiological rhythms. Experimental data supplied by Levine and his associates are extremely encouraging in this respect.

> If one examines the nature of the response of the infant to the surrogate, one sees very clearly differences between the surrogate-reared infant's response to its surrogate and loss of its surrogate when compared to the response of mother-reared infants. A recent experiment (Hennessy, Kaplan, Mendoza, Lowe, & Levine, 1979) indicates that, in contrast to mother-reared infants, the removal of the surrogate from the home cage resulted in a significant increase in behavioral agitation, but under no circumstances did the infant exhibit a change in plasma cortisol levels. . . . Here we have indications of behavioral distress with no indications of physiological arousal. (Levine, 1982, p. 47)

3. As we all know, the distinction of roles between parents is quite specific in Western culture. Social, economic and cultural factors, although somewhat changing today, in addition to the biological factors (pregnancy, breast-feeding, etc.) make the mother–child relationship a closer one than the father–child relationship. Recently, however, there has been growing awareness that the father's role has manifold, pervasive influences on the child's developing self-knowledge. However, these influences may be less appreciable, because as a rule they appear to be more indirect and mediated as compared to the mother's (Biller, 1974; Lamb, 1976; Lynn, 1974). This is why Lewis and Weinraub (1976) have suggested that the father's role should be examined under three major headings.

a. *How the father is described when he is absent.* For instance, comments on the father's success or lack of unsuccess in his job, or his attitude toward the various ups and downs in life, give the child information on what characterizes masculinity, on how he/she should behave as an adult, on what dangers he/she needs to look out for, and so forth.

b. *The quality of the mother–father relationship.* The emotional support that the father offers to the mother is an important observation upon which the child may elaborate beliefs and expectations on the nature of affective relationships. In particular, the male child will form rules regarding the masculine role in the affective relationships (subsequently following them or rebelling against them, according to the quality of his emotional relationship with his father); whereas the female child will form rules on what she can expect from a man in an affective relationship, establishing thereupon a first "draft" of her future approach–avoidance strategies toward males.

c. *The father's observable interaction with the family's social network.* This interaction will allow the child to draw a whole series of rules on how to act in social relationships and how to face the outside world.

4. Without the pretense of offering a complete picture of the distorted identification processes that interfere with adolescent search for an affective autonomy, I shall outline some of the most frequent patterns found in therapeutic practice.

a. *Precarious identification with the homologous parent* (because of his/her relative or absolute absence, and lack of alternative models). Although this situation does not inevitably influence heterosexual adjustment, the capability of adapting to conjugal life and to stable affective relationships seems adversely affected by it. For instance, a male can have difficulties in structuring roles such as husband and father, while masculinity, for him, tends to coincide with heterosexuality (i.e., with sexual performances paralleled by superficial love affairs). Biller (1974) observed that male teenagers with dominant, overprotective mothers and an absent father figure easily took the initiative with girl friends and were usually successful in establishing flirting relationships, but tended to withdraw promptly whenever the flirt seemed to change into a more enduring relationship requiring a stronger emotional commitment. Their style of affective and sexual behavior somewhat resembled the Don Juan stereotype. Similarly, in the female, while there can be a fairly good repertoire of social techniques bound to heterosexuality, the correspondent roles of wife and mother can be precarious.

b. *Lack of the parent of the opposite sex* (because of premature death, early divorce between parents, rejection, and lack of alternative models). In these cases social skills related to courtship or to heterosexual relationships may appear rather rudimentary. Perhaps more frequently, subjects who have had this kind of experience seem to consider themselves prone to being deserted in future affectional bonds or otherwise destined to loneliness. It is possible to hypothesize that this perceived sense of self stems from both modeling with the remaining homologous parent and the lack of a "testing bench" for ascertaining one's lovableness in heterosexual relationships. These individuals usually appear to be rather passive and withdrawn in their affective relationships or otherwise prone to various kinds of provoking, aggressive behavior toward the partner, which, indeed, makes it very likely that desertion will occur (Hetherington, 1972; Hetherington & Parke, 1979).

c. *Conflicting relationship with the parent of the opposite sex.* An unaffectionate parent of the opposite sex (i.e., an ambivalent, hypercritical, overcontrolling one) makes the development of overall negative beliefs about the opposite sex very likely, particularly so if the conjugal relationship between parents is disturbed. As a consequence, the individual may develop a whole range of problematic affective styles (ambivalence toward significant figures, provocative behavior that appears as soon as positive engagement is established, compulsive search for noncontrolling partners, etc.) depending on the specific aspects experienced in his/her troubled relation with the parent. For this reason, such aspects will have to be reconstructed case by case through an accurate developmental analysis of the family's patterns of attachment.

CHAPTER FIVE

ORGANIZATION

Yet the self is a problem and puzzle to itself. A theory should explain
both the self's special awareness and its continuing mystery, even to
itself. —Nozick (1981)

The purpose of this chapter is to outline a descriptive model of
general adult cognitive processes—that is, a conceptual framework
that illustrates how all of the elements comprising a human cognitive
system (tacit and explicit processing, patterns of self-awareness,
etc.) are arranged in a defined organizational relationship endowed
with a self-referent logic. This self-referent organization enables
any individual, through the assimilation of ongoing experience,
to undergo continuous transformations of their perceived sense
of reality without losing his/her unique identity.

For a more systematic exposition, this chapter will consist of
two parts; the first describes the levels and processes characterizing
a human knowing system, while the second discusses the way in
which these levels and processes acquire *systemic coherence*, that
is, work together in an overall personal, cognitive organization.

A TWO-LEVEL MODEL OF KNOWLEDGE PROCESSES

Selfhood processes can be regarded as a coalition of an ordered
range of *explicit* self-images elaborated out of an oscillating array
of *tacit* self-boundaries. Therefore, the developed human cognitive
system includes a higher, tacit organizing level composed of basic
ordering processes. From these the lower, explicit level elaborates
a moment-to-moment and coherent perception of reality, based
upon the data actually available from the upper level and on the
actual environmental influences at that moment. Needless to say,
the two levels are so closely embedded and widely overlapping

in any aspect of mental processing that it would be almost impossible to analyze them separately. Therefore, treatment that follows, as well as Figure 5-1, only conform to a necessity for clearness in the exposition.

The Tacit Organizing Level

This is the higher level of knowledge elaboration in a human cognitive system. Tacit knowledge can basically be regarded as hierarchically arranged clusters of emotional schemata and the deep rules through which they are structured. These deep rules order the ensemble of emotional schemata in differentiated recursive loop that oscillates between opponent boundaries of meaning and organizes the flow of ongoing experience into specific processing patterns.

This superordinate level is the result of a rhythmic differentiation from an interplay between evolutionary and developmental variables. As we have seen, Hayek's (1952, 1978) evolutionary primacy of the abstract (i.e., sensory decoding rules, match-to-pattern process by opponent regulation, self-reference, etc.) accounts for the emer-

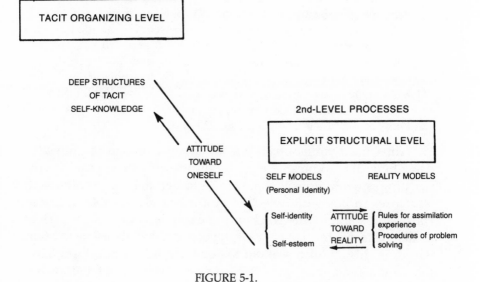

FIGURE 5-1.

gence of human dimensions of consciousness. Constrained by such a structural frame of reference an individual, throughout development, constructs his/her own "ontological" primacy of the abstract (i.e., Tomkins's [1978] ensemble of nuclear scripts). This, in turn, makes possible the emergence of a highly personalized stream of consciousness within the already established dimensions of human self-awareness. Each person, therefore, is at any moment endowed with a personal experiencing of reality that is part of a shared social construction of the world based on invariant, and therefore common, dimensions of meaning.

For a particular individual, this idiosyncratic perception of the world determines to a large extent the very form that each experience will assume, giving consistency and continuity to his/her ongoing feeling of oneness and uniqueness. Tomkins's (1978) account of a man whose tacit boundaries were oscillating between helplessness and anger, as a developmental result of a disrupted deep attachment to his mother, is a very good example in this regard:

> A man is driving his automobile on a lovely spring day on a brand new just-opened interstate highway. He looks at the lush greenery all about him and at the shiny, white new highway. An unaccustomed peace and deep enjoyment seizes him. He feels at one with beautiful nature. There is no one else. He is apparently the first to enjoy this verdant and virginal scene. Then, as from nowhere, he sees to his disgust a truck barreling down the road, coming at him and entirely destroying the beauty of the setting. "What is that truck doing here?" he asks himself. He becomes deeply depressed. He can identify the apparent reason, but he senses that there is more to it—that his response is disproportionate to the occasion, and the depression is deep and enduring. . . . He characteristically does not know why he feels as he does. . . . He is victimized by his own high-powered ability to synthesize ever-new repetitions of that same scene without knowing that he is doing so. (pp. 230–231)

Thus, the rhythmic oscillation between tacit boundaries provides something like a kinesthetic sense of oneself whose implicit felt meaning is continuously explicated into definite representational structures through the selective processing of available ongoing cues—for example, the truck in the example quoted above. This ability rests on the tacit level's responsiveness to its very own decoding rules, which scaffold the ongoing inflow of information into feelings and emotions. Hence, in view of the close relationship between tacit knowledge, emotions, and meaning, we can confidently assume that unconscious processing—via the "collative" effect of patterned ensembles of emotional schemata—corresponds invariably to personal meaning activation (Van Den Berg & Eelen, 1984; Weimer, 1974, 1977). As a consequence, we may further assume that the quality of an individual's consciousness is, at least in part, a function of certain aspects of his/her ongoing tacit oscillating boundaries.

It must be specified that the structuring of tacit knowledge, although acquiring a more defined form during adolescence and youth, does not conclude following this period of maturation. (This notion stands in contrast to the prevailing opinion of traditional psychoanalysis that regards adulthood merely as an endless, passive repetition of earlier developmental themes.) Even after adolescence and youth, the progressive, articulation of deep boundaries— through the production of novel schemata (which interconnect preexisting knowledge structures with incoming information)— stabilizes an ever-changing world by these few invariant principles. As the above example shows, the psychological magnification resulting from the match between one's sense of identity and present experience allows the patterned ensemble of nuclear scripts to grow indefinitely along the individual lifespan. Hence, the most striking feature of the tacit level is certainly its ability to progressively elaborate new frames of reference (i.e., more and more abstract tacit rules) for their subsequent insertion and manipulation into an individual's explicit representations of self and world (Airenti, Bara, & Colombetti, 1982a, 1982b; Guidano, 1984, in press; Welwood, 1982).

The multifold ability to differentiate new emotional schemata is essentially based on the decentralized control that characterizes the tacit level. In other words, the activation of an emotional schema can result just from the differential stimulation of *one* of its constituent processes (e.g., perception, imagery–memory mechanism, visceral–muscular reactions). Additionally, this constituent process, acting upon the entire perceptual structure, may determine a new set of relations among elements of the schema. On the other hand, this activated component, being just an element of an oscillating recursive loop, is immediately integrated into the overall functioning of the entire system. Thus, the particular activated process (e.g., perception) reverberates and automatically spreads over other constituents, such as memory and motor activity. As a result of increasing amplification, the activation may spread to the components of similar but different emotional schemata, reaching so high a threshold as to emerge into one's consciousness (Collins & Loftus, 1975).

The decentralized control of the tacit level, therefore, considerably affects the ongoing experience of reality by bringing into the perceived personal identity feelings, images, and motor patterns that the subject often is not aware of, but that actually change his/ her attitude toward reality. In this way, an individual's tacit apperceptive scaffolding, being the result of a coalition of rather autonomous subprocesses, is much more articulated and expansive than conscious focal attention. For instance, retrieval through the "emotional-memory" mode that tacitly attunes past experiences to current ones, can "per se" allow the articulation of unique aspects of a perceived situation (Bransford, McCarrell, Franks, & Nitsch, 1977). Pylyshyn (1981a) has penetratingly remarked that the relative autonomy of imagery makes the mind faster than even the mind's eye, and that floating intuitions affect our commitments toward significant problems long before they are explicated into plausible representations. Similarly, motor activity and perception of bodily changes, being a special class of amplified perceptions of inner states, can create—via spreading activation—new sets of relations in the ensembles of emotional schemata underlying our sense of identity. This explains why even accurately planned actions can influence our self-perception in a totally different way than had been expected at the moment of performance.

I may conclude by saying that tacit decentralized control— that which makes it possible for us to perceive more than we experience, and to experience more than we attend to (Dennett, 1978)—should be regarded as the basic "push-and-pull" of a human knowing system, constantly making available new sets of tacit relations to be explicated in conscious representation of self and world.

The Explicit Structuring Level

This is a set of explicit models of self and reality stemming from the core schemata of the tacit level and produced by imaginal (Lang, 1979; Pylyshyn, 1973, 1981a) and verbal (Johnson-Laird,

1984; Johnson-Laird & Bara, 1984) thought procedures based upon incoming experience.

With the attainment of analytical skills and reflexive thought, the human knowing system shifts toward a corresponding level of reflexive self-reference and begins to cast the emergent reflexive dimension of consciousness into correspondent patterns of self-awareness—that is, into a stable temporal dimension of reality no longer as critically dependent upon the ongoing decoding of immediate experience as it was during prior stages of cognitive development. Owing to its moment-to-moment ability to integrate one's remembered past, perceived present, and anticipated future into a personal space–time dimension, consciousness unfolds into an ongoing self-synthesized view that provides unity and continuity to the individual's coalition of subprocesses.

Compared to the holistic, immediate, and more abstract tacit level of knowledge organization, conscious representational models give a limited and more incomplete image of self and world. In other words, *not all* the knowledge contained in the tacit level is used in building explicit models, nor is the knowledge content pertaining to ongoing models of self and reality represented in the stream of consciousness with all its details and at every moment. Though represented each time in an episodic way—depending on individual needs and the events that an individual is experiencing—explicit knowledge generally fits the tacit knowledge level on which it depends, with minimal incongruities.

Personal Identity

Tacit self-knowledge is expressed at the explicit level by an ordered set of representational models perceived by the subject as his/her ongoing range of actual and potential self-images. From this arrangement of beliefs, memories and thought processes about the self, an ongoing, self-synthesized, and coherent personal identity emerges.

The perception of a many-sided self is indeed a pervasive and crucial feature of our experiencing life. Each one of us not only has different perceptions and evaluations of ourself in relation to different domains of experience—work, private life, social life, and so on—but also, within each domain, experiences changes in the sense of self according to the quality and intensity of the ongoing emotional experiences. Each of these self-images, in turn, is simultaneously experienced both in the present and in the anticipated future, for example, the potential or "ideal" self-images.

Personal identity, therefore, rather than being a defined entity or a superordinate concept, is like an ongoing process whose recursive nature gives functional unity and historical continuity to the individual coalition of self-subsystems. Due to this integrative capacity, the individual, at any moment and according to particular environmental influences, has a perceived identity that represents merely a single example of his/her range of possible self-images. Furthermore, each self-representation is always perceived as a global experience. This is because conscious focal attention selectively amplifies the working self-structures, while at the same time, inhibits others from rising to active awareness (Posner & Snyder, 1975).

> Who we are and what we experience from one moment to the next are not unilaterally determined by a single reigning "executive self," but are the dynamic product of ongoing competitions among versatile subprocesses. We are, in other words, the moment-to-moment expressions of an unknown number of competing personal realities. (Mahoney, in press).

This coalitional control of explicit models of self—reflecting at the conscious level the decentralized control of tacit processes—supplies the individual with a cognitive flexibility and behavioral plasticity that increases his/her possibilities of adapting to an ever-changing reality (cf. Markus & Nurius, 1986). In fact, the simultaneous activation of competing self-images allows the one self-image that has been sufficiently magnified by the characteristics of the perceived situation to become instantiated, temporarily taking control of the individual's conscious focal attention. The continuous changes of the equilibrium between competing self-images modify the ongoing evaluation of one's perceived identity, creating different self-role enactments inside the same dimension of experience.

Furthermore, explicit decentralized control allows the coexistence of dissimilar and incompatible self-images. These images may be activated in a differentiated way and similarly "disengaged" at different times during a particular temporal sequence. Consider, for example, an individual whose experiencing of a given situation is centered on a well-balanced oscillation between opponent self-images that comprise the "one-up" and "one-down" role in a significant relationship. The subject can, to some extent, keep under control a threatening feeling of discrepancy by continuously shifting from a submissive to a dominant attitude, and vice versa, in the same interactional context, regardless of significant variations of ongoing experience. An oscillative equilibrium can thus be achieved by temporally dislocating opponent self-images whose integration would otherwise require a more demanding rearrangement of the subject's personal reality. In any case, the many-sided nature of the self allowed by explicit decentralized control is usually kept inside certain limits—specific and different from person to person, which helps to maintain an ongoing sense of oneness and historical continuity. Any interruption of our personal identity is invariably experienced as a loss of the very sense of reality, undoubtedly the most disrupting and devastating emotion that any human being can feel.

Personal identity, therefore, represents the basic structure of reference and constant confrontation by which every subject becomes able to monitor and evaluate him/herself in relation to ongoing experience. A structured self-identity, in particular, provides a set of basic expectations directing the individual's patterns of self-perception and self-evaluation, consistent with the selected self-image. The degree of congruence existing between beliefs about one's value on the one hand, and estimates of one's own behavior and emotions on the other corresponds to the degree of self-acceptability and self-esteem. Therefore, self-esteem implies the "theory of emotions" to which one adheres in the relationship one establishes with oneself. This theory defines the range of emotions that one can recognize as one's own, the way one labels and controls them, and the circumstances and ways in which one can express them. Consequently, only feelings belonging to the selected emotional range will be properly decoded and experienced as emotions, while unrecognizable feelings are likely to be experienced as externally caused, "strange" phenomena. Izard (1977) incisively remarked that emotion can exist in consciousness independent of cognition; that is, to *experience* anger and to *cognize* anger are two different phenomena. Theoretical and clinical implications of these remarks shall be discussed throughout the book.

Models of Reality

The range of possible self-images is paralleled by a range of potential representational models of the world distributed along a continuum oscillating between corresponding boundaries of meaning. For example, a person having a range of self-images oscillating between a weak/fragile and a strong/controlled sense of his/herself most certainly will have a perception of reality respectively alternating between an image of a dangerous world in which he/she needs protection, and an image of a reliable world that can be faced in total freedom. In other words, perceived personal identity activates a corresponding specific image of reality that fits the actual, "dominant" self-image with minimal incongruities. Thus, any shift of the "weak–strong" continuum underlying self-perception will be paralleled by a corresponding shift in the "dangerous–reliable" continuum underlying world perception.

Therefore, the ongoing construction of reality models, though biased by tacit self-boundaries, is constantly regulated by personal identity structures so as to build representational aspects of the outside world consistent with interactional attitudes toward reality defined by the particular self-image enacted. This regulating activity is carried out mainly by controlling the executive procedures of the basic set of rules upon which rests the coherence and stability of reality models.

1. Rules that coordinate the assimilation of experience: those that determine which domains of experience are to be held as significant and the patterns of integration of these experiences within preformed knowledge structures.
2. Rules that coordinate problem-solving procedures: different types of logical problem-solving procedures (Bara, 1980) employed in defining both the nature of significant problems and the strategy for dealing with them.

It is important to emphasize that models of reality are the individual's *only* possible means of establishing a relationship with the outside world. In other words, a human knowing system cannot discriminate between external events and their inner representation (Airenti et al., 1982b). Because any imaginative procedure works on data that are consistent with deep, tacit knowledge organization, models of reality depict not only the actual perceived world but in fact *any possible* "imaginable" world.

Attitudes toward Oneself and Reality

The essential feature of the model described thus far involves viewing the different structural levels of knowledge as organized in an overall feed-forward relationship and having feedback systems of control. While tacit self-knowledge invariably biases the temporal progression of knowledge processes, structured personal identity appears to be the main regulator of the whole process. Indeed, as shown in Figure 5-1, any new set of deep relations can be inserted and manipulated in reality models and therefore becomes an effective way of interacting with the world—only *through* personal identity structures. Thus, the level of self-awareness reached is an essential variable that regulates the possibilities of representing more abstract, challenging deep structures and influences to a large extent the quality of knowledge levels set forth by forward oscillative processes. It should be noted (see Figure 5-1) that the controlling function exercised by personal identity is carried out through two basic structural relationships.

Attitude toward Oneself

This defines the ongoing relationship between the explicit self-image and tacit self-knowledge. It essentially consists of a set of feedback systems of control that constrain the individual's access to his/her tacit self-knowledge depending on the level of self-awareness. Such constraints make it possible for the individual to hold contradictory self-images and/or to have models of reality that are only effective within certain very narrow domains. Evidence from many sources relating to self-encoding processes suggests that in the ongoing match between tacit self-knowledge and personal identity, a person has virtually unlimited access to past or current information about themselves, and that the person sets the limits of retrieval (Bower & Gilligan, 1979; Mancuso & Ceely, 1980; Markus, 1977; Rogers, Kuiper, & Kirker, 1977).

Hence, thought processes concerned with self-image primarily depict selective ways of processing internal information rather than the tacit self-knowledge that directly affects us. As a consequence, we cannot expect introspection to be like a "window" open on deep tacit processes, but rather on a biased model of them. Therefore rather than being a more or less reliable "objective self" seen from outside, individual self-awareness corresponds to a continuous process of allocation of one's attention and intention aimed at stabilizing and further expanding the actual experiencing of reality.[1]

In this perspective, the unreliability of verbal reports of one's mental events claimed by Nisbett and Wilson (1977) is no longer tenable. According to recent evidence (Ericsson & Simon, 1980; Miller, 1981; White, 1980), only information in conscious focal attention can be verbalized—that is, information mainly pertaining to the actual, explicit self. Information thus appears in focal attention not in an automated fashion but under the execution of cognitive control; it reflects those processes actively involved with solving unfamiliar problems and successfully adapting to new situations. In this sense, verbal reports provide much useful data about the processes the person is executing to integrate his/her perceived identity with ongoing experience.

Established patterns of attitude toward oneself also largely influence the relationship between the individual's whole organization and his/her ongoing level of awareness. Therefore, within a systems/process-oriented approach verbal reports can give essential information to the therapist for the reconstruction of the client's attitude toward him/herself that, in turn, will have a direct bearing upon the planning of any therapeutic strategy.

Attitude toward Reality

This defines the ongoing structural relationship in which personal identity interacts with incoming experience, making one's plans and behavior consistent with the quality of the attitude toward oneself that has been structured thus far. The structuring of an attitude toward reality, therefore, is hierarchically dependent on the structured attitude toward oneself; in other words, our way of seeing reality—and ourselves inside reality—essentially depends upon how we see and conceive of ourselves. In this way, our models of reality are provided with stability and coherence in an ever-changing world.

The tendency to maintain one's own conceptions of the world is not solely a function of confirmatory-biasing tendencies in reasoning and problem solving (Mahoney & DeMonbruen, 1977;

Wason, 1977). Idiosyncratic problem-solving strategies also permit one to actively manipulate environmental situations so as to produce events that are in keeping with one's perceived identity. Swann and Read (1981), in concluding the discussion on their experimental data, cogently remark: "Through such processes, people may create—both in their own minds and in the actual environment—a social reality that verifies, validates and sustains the very conceptions that initiate and guide these processes" (p. 371).

THE NOTION OF PERSONAL
COGNITIVE ORGANIZATION

The whole is more than the sum of its parts, it is the organizational
closure of its parts. — Varela (1976a)

"Personal Cognitive Organization" (P.C.Org.) refers to the specific organization of personal knowing processes that gradually emerges in the course of individual development. Each individual, though living in an "objectively" shareable social reality, actively constructs at a higher level of perceptual experience his/her own and uniquely private view from within. The most important defining features of a P.C.Org. are its temporal evolution and plasticity—in particular, its ability to undergo changes during the lifespan (sometimes quite radical in nature) and yet continue to maintain a stable sense of oneness and historical continuity.

In the final section of this chapter I shall attempt to frame the relationship between invariance and changeability of a P.C.Org. within a systems approach to complexity, and subsequently to exemplify the dynamic of change that such a viewpoint implies.

Organizational Closure and Structural Openness

The capability of a P.C.Org. to order incoming experience into selfhood structures is at the core of both its autonomy and its invariance as a system. Basically this process involves a form of autonomous computation that, because of its self-referentialness, is considered organizationally closed (Jantsch, 1980; Pask, 1981; Varela, 1979). As previously suggested, in fact, the tacit array of nuclear scripts (e.g., emotional schemata and rules for managing them) is a circular concatenation of apprehensional processes whose coherence lies in their rhythmical recursivity and whose logic is based on self-reference.

On the one hand, because an individual's tacit array of recursive loops rhythmically closes upon itself in arranging the ongoing inflow of experiential data, he/she is able to scaffold experience according to the same, continuous polarities of meaning that his/her very sense of self rest upon. One could also view the autonomous computation entailed by a P.C.Org.'s closure as an "epistemological" constraint; that is, reality itself becomes meaningful (transformed into experience) only if it is processed inside these polarities. On the other hand, throughout a P.C.Org.'s temporal becoming, its organizational closure subordinates the coalition of subprocesses and the pressures for structural changes to the maintenance and further articulation of its tacit self-boundaries (systemic invariance).

In other words, the notion of organizational closure corresponds—no more no less—to the notion of the primacy of the "ontological" abstract in a P.C.Org. The developmental array of nuclear scripts provides a personal experiencing of reality that, after the adolescent symmetry-breaking process, shifts knowledge processes toward the elaboration of a personal, abstract metascript (Abelson, 1981; Tomkins, 1978) or life program (Piaget, 1972). Thus, one's experiencing of reality is now projected into a manipulatable future bringing about a true conception of life, with ethical values, philosophical principles, and metaphysical assumptions. These life-span transformations of the individual's way of experiencing his/her tacit boundaries can be perceived as personal changes inasmuch as they are constantly matched to what in him/her remains unchanged, namely, the rhythmic recursivity between boundaries upon which rests his/her very sense of oneness and historical continuity.

One can, therefore, argue that any P.C.Org., through the organizational closure of its tacit level and the structural openness of its explicit one, is endowed with both a coherent identity and the dynamic transformations that are essential to its continuous viability. Thus, while the organizational closure becomes the very criterion of stability of a P.C.Org., the structural openness of its explicit level, because of its inherent interactions and exchanges, furnishes a generativeness and productiveness to the whole organization (Morin, 1977, 1981; Pask, 1981; Varela, 1976a, 1981).

Therefore, organizational closure and structural openness, rather than being antagonistic, are an expression of opponent regulation processes; the organizational closure of the tacit level, being an abstract self-referent law that constrains the becoming of a P.C.Org., takes place only within a definite space–time dimension and through the specific explicit models of self and world that it can generate.

Thus, the basic "push-and-pull" underlying the directionality of any individual lifespan seems to be the process of making the tacit explicit, whereby individual patterns of organizational closure are further elaborated and articulated in conscious models according to ongoing experience (Davidson, 1980; Guidano, 1984, in press; Welwood, 1979, 1982). Making the tacit explicit should not be viewed as a simple verbal and imaginal translation of deeper level knowledge onto a monitor; on the contrary, it entails an actual *constructive* process—that is, a molding of tacit processes into analytical–analogical thought procedures by the furniture of experience.

This human quest for awareness, rather than being a culturally determined philosophical imperative, seems to be one more epistemological constraint that further distinguishes the autonomous computation of the human mind from the mind of other primates (Bickhard, 1980; Gallup, 1977; Mahoney, in press; Passingham, 1982). Conscious, explicit structuring, in fact, emancipates tacit knowledge from the immediacy of experience and transforms it into concepts (e.g., into something that can be manipulated as objects) thereby extending it to a full range of actual and potential problems. The assimilation of experience produced inevitably leads to an increase of the individual's internal complexity that, in turn, facilitates the further production of new tacit rules for their subsequent insertion into conscious models.

Since the articulation of tacit rules may contribute to the further development of the individual's tacit dimension, the process of making the tacit explicit brings about the potential function of generating self-maintained positive feedbacks leading to even more complex and integrated models of self and world. Keeping in mind the primacy of tacit self-referent logic in the scaffolding of experience, it is possible to consider the increase of complexity that characterizes the orthogenetic progression of an individual lifespan as a series of self-transcendent leaps. In other words, the ever-growing tacit array of nuclear scripts is continuously reelaborated and explicated in light of new experiences that change peripheral and contingent causal theories to more central and integrated ones, thus increasing the subject's feeling of uniqueness and historical continuity. Therefore, it may be concluded that the heuristic possibilities of an individual's tacit level—which, in turn, largely depend on its organizational closure pattern—constrain the set of worlds that are conceivable for that particular individual as well as the range of all his/her possible subjective experiences.

Change and Systemic Coherence

In the perspective described, a P.C.Org. appears as a complex system whose generativeness and productiveness are on the one hand, based on the interplay between organizational closure and structural openness; and on the other, are expressed through a dynamic, progressive equilibrium that, according to the orthogenetic principle, moves toward more integrated levels of structural order and complexity. As noted earlier, the principle underlying the dynamic equilibrium of the lifespan is called "order through fluctuations"; emerging higher-order patterns are the expression of the integration of disequilibriums—or fluctuations—arising out of the ongoing assimilation of experience (Brent, 1978b, 1984; Jantsch, 1980; Mahoney, 1982; Nicolis & Prigogine, 1977; Prigogine, 1976; Weimer, 1983).

The classic notion of stability implies the achievement of a circular, homeostatic equilibrium around an optimum point of reference, through which the system has a constant tendency to return if disturbed by perturbations. Conversely, in a systems approach, a P.C.Org., by restructuring its ordering processes, constantly moves toward other points of equilibrium with the intent of assimilating challenging pressures without altering its adaptative logic. Stability, therefore, is not to be found in a defined "optimal" situation achieved or yet to be achieved, but rather in a dynamic process of *systemic coherence*. Consequently, it will be impossible ever to reach something like absolute stability, just as it will be impossible to identify in an individual lifespan the absolute, optimal situation.

The assertion that a P.C.Org. exhibits a "good" stability at any point in time implies that the individual functions in his/her specific way with fluctuations around a particular reference (Dell, 1982).

Should a fluctuation become amplified to such an extent that it goes outside the individual's existing range of stability, the disequilibrium that emerges will help drive the P.C.Org. in the direction of restructuring its ordering processes. Again, the individual's mental functioning appears to have a generative and endless directionality—not of a linear kind—but rather of a type that might be called the capacity for "continued ongoingness" (Dell & Goolishian, 1981).

What is the nature of the fluctuations upon which the ongoingness of a P.C.Org. is based? As proposed earlier, accessible tacit processes are converted through thought procedures into representational models that constitute the only way one has of understanding reality. As a result of the ongoing tacit ordering of experience, new sets of tacit rules are discontinuously emerging to be subsequently inserted into conscious models. However, if the emergence of new sets of tacit rules represents a challenging and generative possibility for the reorganization of conscious models of self, the outcome of such a deep pressure depends on the integrative capabilities of such models, since they exert a regulatory control on the overall individual organization during its temporal becoming (Epstein, 1973; Greenwald, 1980; Mahoney, 1982, in press). In order to allow any consistent degree of modification of conscious models of self, individuals must gradually modify their self-decoding patterns without experiencing interruptions in their ongoing sense of subjective continuity.

The temporal becoming of a P.C.Org. can therefore be regarded as a history of conscious model changes in relation to the invariance of its tacit-level organizational closure. This invariance–change complementarity (Varela, 1979) unfolds into a temporal dimension through the opponent process regulation between maintenance and change. Actually, these are interplaying and overlapping processes that, though simultaneous, exhibit different modalities during the temporal becoming of a P.C.Org.; *while maintenance processes are continuous, change processes are continuous only as challenges or possibilities, but are discontinuous in their occurrence.*

The Dynamics of Personal Change

Challenging pressures produce different effects on the integrative capabilities of the self, according to their unique qualities and corresponding intensity.

A pressure that is appreciable but contained within the range of stability will produce a reorganization of the person's attitude toward reality without any significant change in personal identity; a person may modify his/her way of understanding aspects of reality without having to change his/her sense of self. These *surface changes* (Arnkoff, 1980; Mahoney, 1980, 1982), though variable according to their intensity and the outcomes they produce, occur continuously and foster endless revisions of conscious models according to ongoing experience. The perception of this type of change is recognizable to the experiencing subject because this process is primarily carried out under cognitive control, and, therefore, within conscious focal attention. As a consequence, the subject can construct explanations and causal theories, no matter how inaccurate, for his/her change (Nisbett & Wilson, 1977), although the individual is sometimes surprised by its suddenness. Surface changes, therefore, are an expression of the level of flexibility and plasticity reached by a P.C.Org. by means of its coalitional control over the subsystems from which it is structured.

In contrast to surface changes, *deep changes* have an entirely different significance. In every case they represent the expression of a modification of perceived personal identity elicited by a challenging deep pressure whose intensity and quality is such that it oversteps the existing stability range. Deep change processes—ranging from a limited restructuring of personal identity to true "personal revolutions" (Mahoney, 1980)—correspond to changes in patterns of attitude toward oneself as a result of the reconstruction of sets of deeper rules emerging from tacit self-knowledge.

The deeper rules appear in the subject's mental processing in the analogical code with which tacit knowledge is generally expressed. Therefore, they essentially take the form of nonverbal and emotionally charged representations (images, fantasies, dreams, sudden recollections, etc.) phenomenologically experienced as unexpected and fleeting "intuitions" (Pope & Singer, 1980; Singer, 1974). Such content may more or less reverberate in the individual's internal representations and initially may not be considered particularly meaningful experiences, especially since they usually assume quite different forms even in a single day.

The tacit processing of such content may proceed to such an extent that some representations begin to appear in an increasingly stable form, and the subject now perceives them as actual "alternative visions" of self and reality. These are to be considered as phenomenal indications of new sets of tacit rules that are reaching the individual sphere of awareness by circumventing one's usual patterns of attitude toward oneself. The duration of the reverberation period and of subsequent, more organized processing, varies widely from case to case. However, even in the more favorable situations, the process is a gradual one and is accompanied by varying degrees of affective distress—the level of which will be more intense the more deeply one modifies the attitude toward oneself.

Since any tacit assumption must pass through personal identity to be introduced into representational models, awareness is a facilitating condition for converting tacit knowledge into beliefs and thought procedures (Airenti et al., 1982a, 1982b). Particularly, the quality of self-awareness—expressed by the corresponding patterns of attitude toward oneself—dramatically influences the shift to a metalevel of knowledge representation and the final result of a deep change process. A deep oscillative process may produce different consequences depending on whether it represents a progressive or a regressive shift in the orthogenetic progression of an individual lifespan.

Progressive shift. The switching to a metalevel of knowledge representation is achieved when processing capabilities, determined by self-awareness patterns, somehow match incoming deep challenges. The structuring of more integrated personal identity allows one to: (1) decode and label the arousal of feelings connected to the deep oscillative process, with a corresponding progressive shift in self-awareness; (2) manipulate even more sophisticated models of reality with a corresponding progressive shift in experience assimilation.

Regressive shift. The switching to a metalevel of knowledge representation is thwarted by a pattern of self-awareness that does not permit the conversion of challenging deep rules into beliefs and thought procedures. The failure to reach a more integrated personal identity has relevant implications from a clinical perspective: (1) The activation of an unintelligible arousal is invariably coupled with the elicitation of negative emotions and unusual perceptions of bodily changes that, in turn, foster the production of erroneous cognitive explanations (Marshall & Zimbardo, 1979; Maslach, 1979). The consequence is a proliferation of external, "ad hoc" theories aimed at explaining overemotionality without altering one's own self-image. This obviously constitutes a regressive shift in self-awareness. (2) Consequently, in spite of unsuccessful predictions and results, reality models become linked even more closely to stereotyped and repetitious imaginal representations and problem-solving procedures, with a corresponding regressive shift in experience assimilation.

In both progressive and regressive shifts, the phase in which the deep oscillative procedure approaches a conclusion is likely to be characterized by a rather abrupt emergence of the individual's different plans and behaviors.

The mechanisms that regulate this sudden emergence are still rather obscure; but are likely to be comparable to Piaget's (1974) "grasp of consciousness" process. Although it is often subjectively identified with an insight that suddenly throws light on aspects of self that up until that moment had remained obscure, this process is, on the contrary, a true construction of something that was being processed and organized at a tacit level for a long time. In other words, only the *act* of becoming aware occurs suddenly; the preceding tacit construction is slow and gradual. One may note that the abruptness and discontinuity that characterizes the "grasping of consciousness" parallel very well the rearrangement of the co-alitional control of a complex system expressed by Thom's (1975) mathematical formalism of "catastrophe theory."

As a further consideration, progressive and regressive aspects are widely overlapping and interdependent in any shift of knowledge levels. Because of a P.C.Org.'s coalitional control, making the tacit explicit is a multilevel and multidirectional process in which different subprocesses are activated with different effects. Whatever kind of integration is attained at the end of a deep oscillative process will invariably contain progressive as well as regressive aspects. Thus, any progressive shift always has its regressive aspects, though obviously secondary. Even the extreme case of the most successful "personal revolution" in which the amount of regressive changes are minimized corresponds to a greater explication of the heuristic possibilities of a P.C.Org., and in the final analysis, to a decrease of its potentialities in the light of its irreversible temporal becoming. Similarly, any regressive shift would also exhibit some progressive aspects, though, for various reasons, they cannot be conveniently employed. As an example, it may be enough to mention the emergent and "creative" capabilities through which an agoraphobic can manage a perceived hostile world. Perhaps no other human being is equipped with such a sophisticated repertoire for the detection and avoidance of imaginable dangers.

It should be quite evident that the temporal becoming of a P.C.Org. is not a continuous, linear process, but rather a discontinuous, step-by-step reorganization. The passage from one step to the next is, in turn, a relatively unpredictable process both in the way it occurs and in the amount of time it takes. As an example, both a "personal revolution"—for example, a successful deep change—and a "clinical syndrome"—for example, an unsuccessful deep change—are simply the expression of different reordering processes elicited by a deep challenging pressure. As Dell and Goolishian (1981) put it: "One can intervene in such systems and push them to the point of instability, but one cannot control precisely when they reorganize, nor can one control in what fashion they reorganize" (p. 179). However, the unpredictability of the human lifespan does not mean, of course, pure indeterminacy, and therefore by no means implies that a person can oscillate randomly between a personal revolution and a clinical syndrome. As shall be suggested in Part 3, the relationship between the whole organization and the ongoing level of self-awareness largely influences the way in which a P.C.Org. will go through a significant fluctuation. In particular, the structured attitude toward oneself—with its specific patterns of selection–exclusion of information—constrains the flexibility of the individual's organizational closure, influencing to a large extent his/her integrative attempts. In other words, the development of an individual lifespan, despite its pattern of uncertainty, is regulated in its unfolding by the systemic coherence belonging to one's specific P.C.Org.

NOTE

1. Since the relationship with our tacit self-knowledge can be only indirect, chances to know ourselves as we really are clearly are just as remote as those of knowing reality in itself. In other words, one can only construct interpretative models of oneself with inferential procedures biased by the same tacit self-knowledge that one would like to know.

The famous words of Socrates, "know thyself," that still bear so much influence on our ethical and philosophical conceptions, can no longer be understood to mean that the ideal goal of an individual lifespan is to succeed in grasping, sooner or later, the ultimate essence of oneself. If we are not completely given to ourselves, then, as Hamlyn (1977) states, "a central fact about self-knowledge is that there is no *thing* to be known" (p. 196). Rather than referring to some specific content of self-knowledge, "know thyself" can only correspond to the moment-to-moment dynamic equilibrium of "being oneself" through a coherent balance between the rational order of our conscious experience and the nonrational dynamics of our tacit boundaries. All the same, even this kind of purpose is bound to remain a regulative–normative ideal, for according to Watts (1958), when human beings acquire the powers of self-awareness and rational thought, they become so fascinated with these new tools that they generally forget ever having used others.

PART THREE

TOWARD A SYSTEMS/PROCESS-ORIENTED PSYCHOPATHOLOGY

CHAPTER SIX

PATTERNS AND PROCESSES

Consciousness and the other higher mental processes are but tools
used by an "I" that cannot be identified with any of them.
—Weimer (1983)

A systems/process-oriented approach to psychopathology can be
regarded as a comprehensive etiological model that attempts to
explain how the unitary interplay between attachment and selfhood
processes may result in specific dysfunctional patterns of attachment.
These patterns may influence the development of certain P.C. Orgs.
that, if destabilized, provide the basic structure for the emergence
of some common clinical syndromes (Bowlby, 1977a; Guidano, in
press; Guidano & Liotti, 1983; Liotti, 1984; Mahoney, in press).
What follows is a detailed analysis of some developmental and
organizational patterns implied by this approach.

THE INFLUENCE OF PARENTING BEHAVIOR ON
DYSFUNCTIONAL PATTERNS OF ATTACHMENT

Because preschool years and childhood represent a gradual disengagement from a condition of almost total complementarity with
parents, parenting behavior during this time is the crucial variable
regulating the quality and course of attachment processes.

The central feature of parenting behavior is the "the provision
by both parents of a secure base from which the child or an adolescent
can make sorties into the outside world and to which he can return
knowing that he will be welcomed when he gets there, nourished
physically and emotionally, comforted if distressed, reassured if
frightened" (Bowlby, 1980b, p. 20). Any limitation or alteration of
the parents' role invariably reflects on the child's developing self-
knowledge and exploratory behavior.

Various psychological conditions can interfere with adequate parenting behavior and these typically reflect the parents' own previous developmental experiences. While forthcoming chapters will examine more closely the dysfunctional patterns of attachment associated with specific P.C.Orgs., at this point the most common sources of problematic parenting behavior will be addressed.

A specific and crucial interfering influence upon an individual's parenting behavior is undoubtedly that person's lack of adequate parental models as a child. Women who, in their childhood, experienced mothering deprivation tend to engage in less interaction with their infants and are less responsive to their children's needs than mothers with happier childhoods (Bowlby, 1980b; Harlow & Harlow, 1965; Harlow, Joslyn, Senko, & Dopp, 1966; Parkes, 1982). Besides the influence of varying degrees of mothering deprivation, it can generally be said that those who have experienced insecure attachments commonly have difficulties in providing a secure base around which their own children can experience a secure attachment to them, as explored by DeLozier (1982): "Since the parents, as children, never had had their own needs met, they were unable to meet the needs of their offspring. This reported breakdown occurred not in the mechanical sense, but in "motherliness," which involves sensitive, empathic interaction with the child" (p. 97).

Another general observation is that a parent's dysfunctional P.C.Org. may interact with specific current life events (marriage, pregnancy, working, life problems, etc.), producing clinical disorders that interfere with parenting behavior. Extensive evidence demonstrates that children of parents with a history of psychological problems are themselves at significant risk of developing psychopathology (Beardslee, Bemporad, Keller, & Klerman, 1983; Cooper, Leach, Storer, & Tonge, 1977; Pound, 1982).

Although any age or stage of development may be affected by inadequate parenting styles, early infancy and adolescence both appear to be crucial phases for different reasons. During infancy, the first stable patterns of self-perception and self-recognition emerge that act as necessary reference points for subsequent matching processes. In contrast, adolescence represents a period of integration that crowns all maturational stages with the establishment of a steady, full sense of personhood.

However, a parenting repertoire limited or altered in any way does not prevent parents from developing an indubitably definite and involving attachment to their children. Parenting behavior is, in fact, one example of a limited class of biologically rooted types of behavior (Bowlby, 1980b). Therefore, the relationship with the child is usually experienced by parents as a central motivation that is matched by a strong urge to behave in certain typical ways, regardless of whether they are up to the task or not. With the same self-referent logic that transforms any basic affective relationship into an identification process, the relationship with the child is likely to be experienced by parents as a central source of potentially available and powerful confirmations to their perceived sense of self. Despite their great variability, upbringing strategies could usefully be considered as an expression of parents' working models of self and reality and of their ongoing identification with the child. The overcontrolling and repressive strategies that we discussed in Shirley's case (p. 74), for instance, clearly represented a father's interpersonal device for obtaining confirmations of his view of himself and the world. The same principle can be applied to those situations representing an "inversion of the parent/child relationship" (Bowlby, 1969, 1973)—exemplified by Derek's case (p. 73). There are data supporting the contention that past unsatisfied need to be nurtured is frequently what leads an abusing parent to seek inappropriate care and reassurance from his/her child (DeLozier, 1982). In some situations, the parent's behavior may be ambiguous and intrusive with little space for intimacy and self-disclosure. Such parents seem to be trying at all costs to give the child an extremely favorable image of themselves, as was the case of Brenda's mother (pp. 60, 62, 75). To consider the child's potential negative judgment as a threat of love withdrawal may be assumed to be another example of a very strong self-confirmatory function attributed to the child.

Though originated by different motivations and sustained by different cognitive abilities, a parent–child relationship can thus be regarded as an extremely complex situation of reciprocal identification. However, the intentions that—consciously or not—inspire parents' upbringing methods only have an indirect influence on the child's developing self-knowledge, because the crux of a parent–child relationship (as far as the influence on the child is concerned) lies in the child's *perception* of what parents are, rather than in their actual attitudes or specific intentions. In other words, it is not the "real" world but how it is construed by the child that has a crucial role in the tacit ordering of his/her personal meaning. Consider for instance, situations in which the child, having witnessed dramatic family scenes, receives pressures from parents to erase them from his/her mind and behave as if they never occurred (Bowlby, 1979, 1985). Although the parents' intention may be one of preserving a positive image of the family, what children may actually experience as a result of the parents' disconfirming behavior is an emergent feeling of unreliability of their own decoding ability that in turn may deeply affect both the further structuring of their self-image and the ongoing identification with their parents.

Reciprocal identification between parents and children, and the consequent reciprocal tacit involvement, are probably at the root of a quite commonly observed phenomenon; namely that, not only may parenting problems be passed from one generation to the next, but so may the attitudes toward oneself and reality ("Generational pattern hypothesis," DeLozier, 1982; Jayaratne, 1977; Kramer, 1985; Merikangas, Leckman, Prusoff, Pauls, & Weissman, 1985; Parkes, 1982). In this reciprocity, because each party identifies with their own perceptions of the other, rather than with the other's real intentions, the dynamics underlying such a generational transmission, like a tangle of endless mirror reflections, seem to elude usual methods of analysis and experimental controls. While still unrecognized as targets for scientific investigation, these dynamics are widely accepted by our "folk psychology" based on the tacit understanding of everyday experience, and are expressed and described mainly in literature and art.

One of Jules Feiffer's cartoons, for example, is poignantly ironical on this subject. It features a woman talking to herself, more or less as follows: "I hated myself for what I'd come to be. . . . That's why I tried to do with my Jennifer the opposite of what Mum did with me. / Mum was possessive, I encouraged independence. Mum was ambiguous and uncertain, while I've been steadfast and determined. Mum was always close and evasive, I was frank and sincere. / Well, the job's done now. Jennifer has grown up. She's Mum's perfect image."

ADOLESCENCE REORGANIZATION AND THE INTEGRATION PROBLEM

In the human species, attachment and contact with parents possess distinctive features that are unprecedented on the zoological scale.

On the one hand, the process goes on for years, usually long after adolescence and youth. On the other hand, in the course of development, attachment becomes a highly structured vehicle through which increasingly complex and exhaustive information about oneself and the surrounding reality becomes available. While children spend a long period of their lives in close contact with their family environment, their parents—guided by their own working models of self and the world—are not likely to change their interpersonal style very much during this time. Therefore, self-knowledge structured since early infancy will develop through constant confirmation because the individual still experiences the same relations that first allowed its definition.

On the threshold of adolescence, the child has reached an actor's sense of his/her perceived self whose emotional and cognitive features have become so engrained that they operate automatically. This arrangement allows one to economize effort by concentrating conscious, rational thought toward specific domains of experience, but also limits the subject's resilience. Since cognition and action have been automated, they are not readily accessible to conscious processing, and so are difficult to modify.

As childhood comes to its end—just at the time when a steady, reliable equilibrium has been attained—the emergence of logical/deductive thinking and the new disequilibrium it implies, urges the subject to seek, through oscillations and uncertainties, a new equilibrium by reorganizing his/her ordering processes. As previously discussed, available abstracting abilities are the crucial ingredients of the adolescent re-equilibration and integration between opponent selfhood processes.

A systems/process-oriented approach to the development of intelligent abstract behavior not only emphasizes the activity of solving conflicts and contradictions as being important to the development of cognitive abilities and self-analytical skills, but also considers the conflicts and contradictions themselves as a fundamental quality of thought and creativity (Brent, 1984; Charlesworth, 1969, 1976; Miller, 1978; Miller & Wilson, 1979; Riegel, 1979). However, if the challenging situation that causes the conflicts is beyond the child's coping abilities, it will limit and distort, instead of promote, the unfolding of cognitive growth. An overwhelmingly challenging situation becomes an inescapable, essential concern to the child's survival. Besides altering the quality of cognitive growth, it concentrates his/her resources on obtaining an adaptative equilibrium with respect to a domain of experience that is too narrow, altered, and therefore, hardly generalizable to other aspects of reality. In other words, the eccessive effort required to adapt to highly critical circumstances reduces the chances of development of the subject's cognitive processing abilities by forcing him/her from the start to "specialize" in too narrow a situation.

In most cases, these situations are related to dysfunctional patterns of family attachment reflecting the peculiarities of the surrounding cultural and social network that limit the rate of a child's intellectual stimulation. Of course it is impossible to find "objective" parameters to establish whether or not a challenging situation can be dealt with and to what degree it may be dysfunctional. The notion of "unbearable stress" therefore, is grounded in the subjective construction of personal experience. Because such dysfunctional situations have important clinical implications, a discussion of the developmental process that can interfere with adolescent integration and the kinds of limitations that may accompany these processes is presented.

Interference with Emerging Abstracting Abilities

The negative impact of dysfunctional patterns of attachment upon the development of a child's self-knowledge is reflected both in the contents of nuclear scripts (losses, rejections, frightening scenes, etc.) and in the intensity of the arousal that usually accompanies their activation. In order to reach an adaptive proximity to attachment figures—remember that the very survival of the child depends on it—an essential strategy consists of controlling the disruptive effects of overemotionality. This is typically accomplished by increasing the defensive exclusion of information and by structuring adequate diversionary activities (see Bowlby, 1980a).

A growing body of evidence suggests that differentiated patterns of decentralized control become operative very early in development. For example, after repeated episodes of separation and rejection, usually by mothers who refuse physical contact and any intrusion of the child into their personal space, infants precociously develop active patterns of visual, physical, and communicative avoidance toward caregivers. Such avoidance can be considered to reflect a specific pattern of decentralized control aimed at maintaining one's behavioral organization, since it allows one to keep the arousal of intense emotions activated by problematic contacts below critical levels, while at the same time maintaining a certain degree of proximity even in the aversive condition of maternal rejection (Main & Weston, 1982). Something similar is reported to occur in abused children who exhibit peculiar behavior characterized by silence, extraordinary stillness, and a fixed gaze, even in a painful situation. This pattern has been termed "frozen watchfulness" (DeLozier, 1982; Ounsted, Oppenheimer, & Lindsay, 1975).

Because critical tacit self-knowledge—marked by patterns of coalitional control similar to those described above—is quite stable and not easy to change, it has a pervasive influence on the childhood match-to-pattern processes. This is because the greater the centrality of the critical nuclear scripts, the greater will be the intensity of affect associated with their confirmation or disconfirmation. More specifically, the oscillation of critical self-boundaries, accompanied by intense affective arousal, interferes with the proper articulation of the interplay between emotional differentiation and cognitive growth throughout childhood, restraining the subsequent processing abilities of adolescent formal thought.

In addition to focusing available cognitive abilities on too narrow and specific domains of experience, the struggle for managing intense feelings restricts the child's possibilities of reaching more articulated levels of concrete abstraction. This first becomes evident in the child's limited *distancing capability*—which decrease his/her potential for elaborating a temporal field beyond the one of direct perception. The child therefore is likely to be plunged into a swift stream of events and be unable to enmesh this flux of activity within an ordered temporal scheme. Another important consequence of this process is a limited *decentering ability,* that is, a low conceptual perspective-taking ability that restricts the child's possibility of differentiating and matching his/her opinions and feelings with those of others. This will further interfere with the capacity to order and decode one's feelings and emotions and, by stabilizing "object-bound" attitudes, will negatively affect the whole ongoing differentiation between self and others.

On the other hand, as noted before, impaired cognitive practice in turn reverses its effects on the emotional level by limiting the articulation of the personal range of decodable emotions. More specifically, ensembles of emotional schemata are transformed less and less into semantic–cognitive content, and such information consequently will be mainly stored, represented, and retrieved through other channels, such as perception, imagery–memory mechanism, and motor patterns. The activation of these emotional schemata has a tendency to be directly expressed through muscular–visceral reactions, and also is likely to be paralleled by the emergence of rather undecodable feelings and images in the stream of consciousness. The restriction of their access into conscious, focal attention (through available patterns of decentralized control based on defensive exclusion and diversionary activities) progressively becomes the child's principal strategy of maintaining the stability of his/her working models of self and reality. This obviously further interferes with the already impaired distancing and decentering abilities.

In other words, since dysfunctional patterns of family attachment usually tend to remain stable in time, a self-perpetuating, positive feedback loop is established, in which cognitive abilities are interfered with and overridden by affective pressures. At the end of childhood, although the child has very often achieved a "good" adjustment to a bad situation, the range of concrete and preformal processing abilities will consequently be restricted and reduced in many ways, while ongoing emotional development will, in turn, be rather undifferentiated and scarcely controllable. These conditions decrease the possibility of conveniently reorganizing the disequilibrium that accompanies the emergence of adolescent formal operations. Formal, abstract thought is, indeed, new in the arrangement it entails, not just in content, and its range of processing abilities, as well as the level of abstraction that can be attained, depend, therefore, on the level of distancing and decentering reached during childhood.

Effects on the Concreteness–Abstractness Dimension of Adolescent Integration

For an adequate comprehension of the effects of dysfunctional patterns of attachment during childhood on the subsequent adolescent reorganization, it is best to first analyze the relevant cognitive operations that a subject must carry out as a response to emerging self-analytical skills; namely, focusing and ordering the contradictory aspects of one's self-perception in such a fashion as to promote their adequate integration later on. In fact, since problems are not given, but are a human construction designed to make sense of complex and challenging situations, the quality of problem setting determines, to a large extent the corresponding quality of problem-solving strategies.

In this regard, reduced abstracting abilities influence formal/logical operations from the time they first begin to appear, favoring a formalization of the emerging contradictory aspects of the self in an exceedingly concrete and, therefore, reductive way. On the one hand, reduced possibilities of distancing and decentering hinder the subject from going beyond the field of perceptual experience and induce him/her to immediately identify the not yet under-standable and controllable aspects of his/her self-boundaries with many unbearable and personally negative traits. Furthermore, be-cause of the persisting object-bound attitude, such inferred negative traits cannot be arranged inside an overall, comprehensive self-image, and are therefore most probably perceived as "concrete," separate entities to be isolated from oneself. On the other hand, the reduced possibilities of decoding and controlling inner states intensify the level of involvement with one's perceived situation, inducing the subject to seek a priori severe, urgent solutions without considering all the possible aspects of the problem.

Through a reconstruction of the personal histories of non-psychiatric and psychiatric subjects, Beattie-Emery and Csikzent-mihalyi (1981) found the psychiatric sample to be significantly more concrete in their formalizing of various personal problems that occurred during adolescence.

> The respondents in the psychiatric sample tended to blame, focus attention on, and place at the center of perception, negative aspects of self or parent. In contrast, persons in the non-psychiatric group, as a whole, tended to put into broader perspective the negative aspects of self and family members, and through the use of mechanisms of abstraction and generalization, tended to transform, perceptually or interpretatively, the personal problems into problems occurring at the generalized level of humankind. (p. 391)

A concrete, summary formalization of contrasting aspects related to the emergent felt dichotomy between a perceived "apparent" self (the way the subject behaves in specific situations) and a per-ceived "real" self (the way in which the subject is affected by his/her deep boundaries apart from the situation's specific aspects) produces, as an almost necessary consequence, an equally concrete and partial integration.

The concrete, object-bound attitude binds the individual to the ongoing cognitive situation. Thus, one considers "real" only those aspects of self that directly originate from that situation and excludes all others as negative or at least interfering with the current adaptation, which is seen as the only possible one. This perspective also forces the subject to respond to emerging cognitive demands as if they were an external situation—accepting passively these insights as nothing less than unavoidable fatalities.

The re-equilibration and integration process between contradictory aspects of self is thus completed with the exclusion from conscious access of the challenging and less controllable aspects of one's self-knowledge. Explicit strategies, however, can by no means prevent a tacit responsiveness to ongoing inflow in terms of feelings and emotional schemata. Consequently, the quality of individual consciousness remains a function of those very aspects intended for exclusion. In turn, the emerging potential range of explicit self-images will contain a rather high degree of contradictions and incongruities still awaiting formalization and integration.

The moment-to-moment self-synthesizing process underlying one's perceived personal identity can at this point maintain a certain degree of stability and coherence provided that, at the same time, a rigid and selectively defensive attitude toward oneself is structured through rather sophisticated mechanisms of self-deception (Gur & Sackeim, 1979; Hamyln, 1974; Russell, 1978). The resulting limited range of competing self-images available both restricts the domains of possible experience and reduces the subject's flexibility and plasticity in these same domains, thus lessening the quality and quantity of experience assimilation.

In other words, even after adolescence—and therefore at a more abstract level—those same self-perpetuating positive feedbacks (in which distancing and decentering abilities are interfered with and overridden by affective pressures) are very likely to repropose themselves. Once again, in spite of the adolescent revolution, the individual remains anchored to patterns for ordering reality typical of immature and primitive thinking. These patterns are characterized by one-dimensionality, globality, invariance, and irreversibility and are replete with inferential errors—polarized thinking, arbitrary inference, overgeneralization, and so on—that have been amply described by Beck (see Beck, 1976; Beck, Rush, Shaw, & Emery, 1979). It should be no surprise to discover that these conscious models of self and world, emerging as a result of the ongoing integration, are very often directly related to subsequent clinical complaints. The examples of Derek's (p. 73), Shirley's (p. 74), and Brenda's (pp. 60, 62, 75) adolescence clearly demonstrate this relationship. Derek's case also shows one of the most frequent mechanisms underlying a maladaptive adult affective style—namely, a more or less direct transposition, in new affective domains, of the same affective patterns developed throughout development. While these patterns may have proved to be effective ways of maintaining proximity in childhood, they often have the opposite effect later in life.

PERSONAL COGNITIVE ORGANIZATIONS AND PSYCHOPATHOLOGICAL PATTERNS

The early developmental array of nuclear scripts, through the unfolding of emotional differentiation and cognitive growth, becomes increasingly articulated into personal meaning—that is, one's way of coding reality so as to find evidence for one's very sense of self and world in everyday experience. At the end of the maturational process, the quality of adolescent integration determines the level of abstractness or concreteness that will be the starting point for subsequent articulation of the personal meaning for the rest of one's life. To summarize what has been discussed thus far, it could be stated that the organizational closure and systemic coherence of a P.C.Org. is expressed by the continuity of an individual's core ordering processes throughout his/her lifespan development.

Now, the central argument that will be developed throughout the rest of this book is that *different patterns of organizational closure—structured on the basis of different specific developmental pathways—correspondingly underlie the expression of different clinical patterns.*

Up to this point in time, psychology has addressed clinical disturbances primarily within a descriptive and dispositional framework whose primary aim has been to reduce the complexity of psychological disturbances into a range of suitable terms and labels (e.g., see the well-known DSM-III). Conversely, a systems/process-oriented approach suggests that the wide individual variations of surface-structure features found in clinical observation can be subsumed under a limited number of deep invariant patterns of organizational closure. According to the quality of ongoing tacit and environmental pressures, surface features are believed to be causally related to these deep patterns of organizational closure. This permits the identification of some specific basic personal meaning organizations whose articulation takes place through the structuring of equally specific, though variable, patterns of self-preoccupation. Clinical experience has permitted the identification of four basic patterns of organizational closure that closely correspond to well-known nosological syndromes—namely, depression, agoraphobia, eating disorders, and obsessive–compulsive patterns (Guidano & Liotti, 1983; Guidano, in press; Liotti, 1984).

In the depressive pattern, early distressing events are elaborated as losses, rejections, and the like. Personal meaning is centered on a sense of loneliness and is organized on a deep, self-recursive loop of emotional schemata and tacit rules oscillating between helplessness and anger.

In the agoraphobic pattern, the developmental interference with exploratory behavior and search for autonomy causes the personal meaning to become organized on a self-recursive loop oscillating between the need of protection from a perceived hostile world and the need for absolute freedom and independence in the same world.

In the eating disorders pattern, the distressing experience of having a stable self-perception only by way of an enmeshed relationship with a beloved figure (i.e., a "loose" demarcation between self and nonself) causes the personal meaning to be centered on a blurred sense of personal ineffectiveness. Thus, personal identity becomes organized around deep boundaries oscillating between the need to be approved by significant others and the fear of being intruded upon or disconfirmed by significant others.

Finally, in the obsessive–compulsive pattern, the developmental elaboration of an ambivalent perceived sense of self (as a result of an equally ambivalent attachment to a significant parent) causes personal meaning to become organized around opponent, antithetic, and dichotomous (positive–negative) oscillating self-boundaries. This organization is manifested by way of a compulsory need to reach absolute certainty in every aspect of experience.

Because each of these patterns of organizational closure is structured around a basic core of oscillating emotional polarities within a recursive loop, the unity and continuity of personal meaning processes is based on the organizational unity of one's *emotional* domain (Marris, 1982). Indeed, the self-recursive oscillation of central emotional polarities provide the decoding context for recognizing and experiencing a wide range of ongoing inner states within a single, coherent, and continuing dimension. Moreover, because the progressive organization of one's emotional domain is carried out by means of the interconnection between feelings, on the one side, and patterns of perceptual, visceral, and muscular responses, on the other, one may legitimately wonder whether a specific pattern of organizational closure is matched by an equally specific pattern of psychophysiological response. An initial series of studies from this perspective have supplied encouraging results in favor of the existence of specific patterns of psychophysiological responses in the four above-listed P.C.Orgs. (Blanco & Reda, 1984).

It should be noted, however, that P.C.Orgs. should not be regarded as separate entities consisting of a number of defined and characteristic knowledge contents (e.g., beliefs). In other words, they are not the equivalent of another purely descriptive set of terms and labels for the classification of common clinical disorders. On the contrary, each one is to be considered as a *unitary ordering process* whose coherence and continuity can be grasped only in the specificity of the formal, structural properties of its knowledge processing, rather than in the definite semantic properties of its knowledge products.

A structural analysis of cognition entailed by a systems/process-oriented approach suggests that a pattern of organizational closure is defined by deep invariant syntactic rules capable of generating a consistent range of surface, semantic representations according to an ever-changing interaction with the world. These rules represent a sort of grammar of cognition that explains why processing, despite the diversity of possible experiences, occurs in its specific way and not in others (Pylyshyn, 1981b; Weimer, 1984). The organizational unity of personal meaning, therefore, determines the kind of systemic coherence to which a P.C.Org. is constrained during its lifespan development. Thus, once one knows the laws of a closure, rather than attempting to make a stimulus–response analysis, one can reasonably predict the compensation for any possible perturbation (Varela, 1976a).

Although the described P.C.Orgs. have proven to be the most typical and frequent in my clinical experience over the last 15 years, this by no means suggests that they can explain all the most common clinical syndromes. Further research and improvements in methodology will undoubtedly reveal other basic personal meaning organizations. I am convinced, however, that there is but a small number of possible basic personal meaning organizations—perhaps within the range of one-digit numbers—and that this reflects the equally small number of fundamental emotions that human consciousness can experience (Ekman, 1972; Izard, 1977, 1980; Plutchik, 1980, 1983).

Finally, although these P.C.Orgs. have been labeled mainly from the viewpoint of the clinical disturbances that they can produce, in my opinion they are present also in normal subjects. As has already been suggested about other mental dimensions, normalcy, rather than being identified with something called "normal" P.C.Org. or "normal" knowledge content, lies in the unfolding of a dynamic process—that is, in the generativity with which a specific P.C.Org. develops its systemic coherence throughout the lifespan, and in the higher levels of organized complexity and self-transcendence that it is consequently able to achieve.

In other words, in a systems/process-oriented approach, as Marmor (1983) has pointed out, "normalcy, neurosis, and psychosis should not be regarded as static and fixed entities but rather as dynamic and changeable states of behavior that are potentially reversible, and the borders of which are often indistinct" (p. 834). Therefore, along the normalcy–psychosis continuum, the same P.C.Org.—depending on the quality and elaboration of developmental experiences—can evolve toward a "neurotic" condition if the concreteness–abstractness dimension is insufficiently articulated, or drift toward a "psychotic" condition if (in addition to the constraint of a concrete computation) there is a more or less stable interference in the self-synthesizing integrative ability that provides functional unity to one's perceived personal identity.

THE DYNAMICS OF COGNITIVE DYSFUNCTION

The essential feature of a P.C.Org. whose adolescent reorganization was completed at a relatively low level of abstracting abilities is a significant degree of discrepancy and incongruity in its tacit–explicit relationship. On the one hand, the individual elaborates explicit models of self and the world based on the exclusion from conscious access of challenging and less controllable aspects of his/her deep boundaries; but, on the other, the quality of individual consciousness remains to some extent a function of those very aspects that he/she intends to exclude. This is because conscious procedures cannot prevent a tacit responsiveness to ongoing inflow in terms of emotional schemata and feeling memories.

A trend of this kind, left to itself, would lead to a sort of disunity of individual consciousness. This can be offset by one's ongoing self-synthesizing ability—provided that the accessibility to one's tacit domain is restricted through the structuring of a deceiving attitude toward oneself. A narrow and rigidly concrete attitude toward oneself usually makes it difficult for an individual to explicate tacit processes, in particular the most challenging ones—that is, the ones that would actually supply the most significant information for a restructuring of current models of self and world according to ongoing experience. For this reason, the narrow-margin equilibrium of such a P.C.Org. can reach critical levels of instability and incoherence whenever it is confronted with the necessity of integrating fluctuations arising from the ongoing articulation and transformation of its personal meaning processes as a result of experience assimilation.

Therefore, a cognitive dysfunction can be regarded as a regressive reordering process elicited by a challenging deep oscillation that does not fit with the ongoing patterns of self-awareness, but has attained so high a level of tacit elaboration that it can circumvent the current self-deceiving attitude toward oneself and exert direct pressure on conscious models. The narrow, object-bound structure of the attitude toward oneself, however, forces an individual to consider "real" only the current aspects of his/her perceived personal identity. Consequently, this makes one experience any oscillation toward a change in self-perception as a loss of one's very sense of reality. In such a situation, there are only two possible directions for reordering processes to move: (1) toward an increasing reduction of conscious access to one's tacit domain, and (2) toward regarding the already emerged tacit data as alien to the self.

The attempt to maintain one's ongoing perceived personal identity against a challenging pressure to revise it, underlies the crucial feature of cognitive dysfunction: a sort of "splitting-up" between tacit and explicit knowledge processes; that is, between one's immediate experience of self and one's conscious attention and cognition. This characteristic feature of the emergence of a cognitive dysfunction can be schematically exemplified with a clinical vignette.

Albert was a 33-year-old engineer who asked for treatment because in recent months he had been experiencing panic attacks during which he experienced a fear of impending madness. For our purposes, it will be sufficient to analyze the onset mechanism of the first panic attack according to the reconstruction obtained through clinical assessment.

Albert's developmental history was characterized by an intense anxious attachment with a rigid, undemonstrative mother (the only figure available for him) that limited his exploratory behavior and autonomy with rigid controls and threats of desertion and love withdrawal. Furthermore, his family's meager financial situation forced him to regard studying as the only possible way to reach an acceptable degree of self-competence and self-worth inside the attachment relationship that defined the limited reference scheme of his particular situation. As a result, he grew up without contacts with peers of either sex, relying only on his mother's support, marked by a low degree of emotional warmth and strong conceptions of duty and obligations. During adolescent reorganization, his past experience influenced him to elaborate a self-image of a rational, logical man without emotions or anything else that could appear as "irrational" or "unpredictable." This view oriented him toward mathematical interests when enrolling at the university. When he started to work for a renowned research institute, he felt convinced that the only goal to be pursued in his life was to become a man made up of only abstract, logical thoughts. "I wanted to be just pure thought," were his words.

Soon after his mother died, Albert—who was accustomed to working alone with the silent support of a female figure in the background—married a rather cold, detached, and passive woman. Long before the first panic attacks, their marital relationship had become completely stagnant. They never had affective and communicative exchanges, and their sexual life, very poor from the beginning, was almost nonexistent. On weekdays, he generally came home late in the evening, having spent the whole day at the research institution where he worked. His wife and children were already in bed, and he usually ate his dinner in the kitchen more or less in the dark because, of course, he felt it necessary to save energy.

One day, while going up to his laboratory with some colleagues the elevator suddenly jammed for 1 or 2 minutes. He did not experience any fear at the time and actually continued to converse with his captive colleagues until the elevator resumed operation. One month later he was eating alone in the kitchen at night and an image of the jammed elevator suddenly appeared in his mind, and at the same time he felt a strong sense of constriction. What frightened Albert more than this unpleasant sensation was the discovery of a comparison he was making in his mind in the form of a question and answer: "What difference is there between the jammed elevator and my home? All things considered, they are very similar. There is no way of getting out of them."

In other words, a set of deep challenging data regarding his affective life had become available to him. Up to that moment, it never had the chance of being converted into a format that he could recognize. In the month that followed the elevator episode, there had apparently been a further tacit elaboration of the reverberating images of the jammed elevator, making them useful cues for scaffolding his emerging feelings. However, the emergence itself of that kind of "irrational" consideration represented for Albert a critical event, since it was unbearable for him to accept that it emerged from his conscious self. The apparent illogicality of comparing his home to an elevator was experienced by Albert as a breakdown of his mental faculties, the evidence that he was about to go insane, that is, irrational and illogic, something he had always equated with death. In that very moment he felt the first panic attack.

This splitting-up between tacit and explicit knowledge processes, prevents the possible decoding of an emerged felt meaning (crucial to the structuring of ongoing perceived aspects of oneself and thus inescapable) and interferes with the self-synthesizing ability based on the inhibitory and amplificatory functions of conscious explicit processes (Posner & Snyder, 1975). This state of affairs produces a stable level of overemotionality. The consequent disequilibrium, in turn, drives the individual to further intensify the ongoing tentative reordering processes aimed at dealing with the discrepant felt meaning by preventing him/herself from becoming fully aware of it.

In this perspective, therefore, the central feature in the dynamics of a cognitive dysfunction consists of the continuous, oscillative interplay between two sets of opponent competing knowledge processes that usually oversteps the range of the individual's possibility to reach a more adaptative integrating balance between them. The two sets of competing processes can be summarized as follows (Guidano, in press; Van Den Bergh & Eelen, 1984).

1. *Processes related to conscious explicit processing centered on the attempt to maintain as much as possible the customary self-image.* These processes are generally carried out along two simultaneous directions.

a. Elaboration of cognitions that deny the very nature of the discrepant felt meaning and allow the subject to experience it as something alien to the perceived nature of the conscious self. In the technological revolution presently transforming Western civilization, the notion of "illness" is becoming more and more the only acceptable explanation, both at the existential and social level, for something that, though felt alien, nevertheless has deep influence on behavior and emotion. As in Albert's case, a multitude of theories and beliefs about disease generally accompanies in these circumstances the subjective appraisal of the emergence of a personal crisis.

b. Elaboration of diversionary activities (Bowlby, 1980a) aimed at reducing the possibility of enacting in the actual environment those competing alternative self-images that are activated by the same discrepant felt meaning and experienced as unbearable frightening challenges. The constriction that Albert had unwillingly experienced in his family life was almost automatically matched by the production of fantasies and images of liberation from marriage. But to Albert, these representations confirmed his impending madness and produced a totally different effect; he felt he was able to control anxiety only when he was with his wife—as if only the formation through diversionary activities of a "wife-bound" attitude could confirm the "unreal" nature of those other floating alternative self-images.

2. *Processes related to unconscious activation of personal meaning meant to revise the customary self-image through a stable assimilation of now available tacit data.* Although the discrepancy with ongoing conscious processes undermines the possibilities of scaffolding the tacit activation into more decodable emotions, the discrepant felt meaning will manifest through a continuous surfacing of emotional outbursts that tend to aggravate the existing disequilibrium. Lacking a proper cognitive mediation, the motor setting that accompanies the activation of intense, uncontrollable feelings has a tendency to be directly realized, the excitation does not meet with any delay

and immediately proceeds to its terminus (Luria, 1976, quoted by Van Den Bergh & Eelen, 1984, p. 196). In Albert's case, for instance, the sense of constriction that accompanied the activation of his discrepant felt meaning was so intense and uncontrollable that it could be immediately elicited (and cause conspicuous anxiety crises) in all those situations in which he could not rely on a quick way of escaping. These situations were therefore felt as unbearable limitations to his freedom of movement (elevators, barber shops, highways, subways, etc.).

The course of cognitive dysfunction can have a variable trend that depends both on the quality of the specific P.C.Org. involved, and on the life events that take place as a response to the arisen disequilibrium.

In some cases the oscillative interplay between competing knowledge processes can in the end lead to an integrated balance, with a resulting progressive shift in the individual's self-awareness. It is obviously the most favorable situation, in which a cognitive dysfunction is merely a manifestation of an existential crisis that will give way to a process of personal growth. In less favorable instances the outcome is the achievement of a sort of paradoxical stable equilibrium capable at least of providing relative control to the ongoing high level of overemotionality. This was the case with Albert; the intensity of initial panic attacks could be better controlled, as soon as his wife-bound attitude became quite stable.

To conclude, it should be specified that, in the temporal course of a cognitive dysfunction, when the oscillative interplay resulting from the splitting-up between knowledge processes becomes so intense as to overstep completely the P.C.Org.'s ongoing self-synthesizing ability, the conditions are posed for the emergence of psychotic disturbances. In other words, in order for a disequilibrated P.C.Org. to maintain its functional continuity, it is necessary that the tendency toward disunity of consciousness (caused by the splitting-up between feelings and thoughts) be constantly brought together within the unity provided by selfhood processes. Weimer's remark given in the epigraph will, at this point, become clear in its full meaning, if we consider that neurosis and psychosis are but different states of systemic coherence—carried out by corresponding different dimensions of reflexive consciousness—that a single P.C.Org. can assume as a function of the self-synthesizing ability inherent to its selfhood processes.

TABLE 6-1

Major features of selected P.C.Orgs. in a clinical sample (N = 270)

Feature	Depression (N = 50)	Agoraphobia (N = 130)	Eating disorders (N = 60)	Obsessive–compulsive patterns (N = 30)
Dysfunctional patterns of attachment	Loss/separation; patterns of "affectionless control"	Overprotective; *indirect* interference with exploratory behavior	Ambiguous, "intrusive enmeshment"	Ambivalent, "double-bind" attachment
Sense of self	Negative self with emphasis on self-reliance	Controlling agent	Blurred and wavering	Antithetical/opposite
Major themes on systemic coherence	Oscillations between helplessness and anger	Oscillations between loneliness and constriction	Oscillations between seeking and avoiding intimacy	All-or-none oscillations between certainty and uncertainty
Common coping strategies	Compulsive self-reliance	Control of self and significant relationships	Seeking supportive intimacy that demands minimal self-exposure	Seeking certainty through systematic doubt

After outlining some of the basic patterns and processes, we can now proceed to a more detailed analysis of the P.C.Orgs. briefly mentioned in this chapter. This study is based on clinical observations on a total of 270 psychotherapeutic relationships, the majority of which the author was personally involved in either as therapist or as supervisor. The composition of the client sample, as well as the most common features of P.C.Orgs. about to be discussed, are shown in Table 6-1.

Because the purpose is to outline the development and organization of each P.C.Org., I shall not provide detailed descriptions of the most common symptoms and clinical pictures. The reader who wishes to go deeper into the subject is referred to a previous work (see Guidano & Liotti, 1983). Similarly, clinical vignettes reported were selected in order to exemplify the *systemic coherence* of personal meaning processes rather than for their actual symptomatologic relevance.

CHAPTER SEVEN

THE DEPRESSIVE COGNITIVE ORGANIZATION

I wouldn't belong to a club that wanted me as one of its members.
—Groucho Marx

The central core of a depressive-prone individual consists of a marked responsiveness to even minimal discrepant life events in the form of helplessness and hopelessness as a result of an active scaffolding of these events in terms of losses and disappointments (Bowlby, 1980a; Brown, 1982; Brown & Harris, 1978; Guidano & Liotti, 1983).

Although the discussion that follows is largely compatible with data offered by current cognitive models of depression (Beck, 1976; Beck, Rush, Shaw, & Emery, 1979; Seligman, 1974, 1975; Shaw, 1979; Shaw & Dobson, 1981), the reader will inevitably notice some relevant differences from them. Such differences are to be attributed to a methodological choice of ordering the avoidable clinical and experimental data into a systems/process-oriented framework. In this perspective, I shall first attempt to outline the developmental and organizational processes underlying the systemic coherence exhibited by a depressive P.C.Org. Second, it will be shown how that same systemic coherence can produce, when disbalanced, those patterns of emotional disorders commonly called depressive disturbances.[1]

DYSFUNCTIONAL PATTERNS OF ATTACHMENT

The central feature of the developmental pathway of depressive-prone individuals is the ongoing elaboration of a sense of loss that parallels the abnormal course of their attachment relationships with parents. Patterns of attachment that can foster the elaboration of loss experiences are of different kinds and can occur in a single individual either separately or in combination with each other. The most common seem to be as follows.

1. *Actual loss of a parent during childhood.* A significant amount of data indicates that there is a fairly high probability that more depressed individuals have experienced the death of a parent before or during adolescence than have psychiatric nondepressed patients (Beck, 1967). Brown and his colleagues (Brown, 1982; Brown & Harris, 1978) studying two groups of women—a patient group and a community group—found that 47% of women who had lost their mothers before the age of 11 were suffering from depressive disorders during the observation period, as compared to only 17% of the remaining women.

Another situation that can be included in the category of actual losses is a final or prolonged separation from a beloved parent while the subject was a child or a teenager. In most cases the separation is due to parents' divorce or to one parent being away from the family for work reasons.

The statistical significance of early loss in adult depression seems to be unquestionably evident; in my own sample of depressive clients, percentages are not significantly different from those reported in the literature. On the other hand, it is quite obvious that not every child who experiences loss or separation from a parent develops depression later in life, even when faced with further serious losses or disappointments. One hardly needs to point out that the processing of a sense of loss—just as any personal meaning elaboration—is an active scaffolding of ongoing experience that has no direct correlation with the quality and intensity of "objective" life events. Therefore, in addition to the objective event of separation, interpersonal cues are necessary to facilitate its structuring in terms of loss. Consider, for example, the case in which parental attempts to obtain control over the child's behavior are mainly carried out through threats of desertion or withdrawal of love. If such threats are subsequently followed by periods of physical separation, they are more likely to be experienced by the child as affective losses provoked in some way by him/herself. In other words, as Rutter (1972, 1979) pointed out, it is not so much the separation itself that has an influence on the child as the quality of the relationship that precedes, accompanies, and follows it.

2. *The experience of never having been able to attain, throughout maturational stages, a stable and secure emotional attachment, despite*

continuous efforts in this direction (Bowlby, 1980a). The most frequent of such situations is one in which parents are uneffusive, apparently detached, and attribute special importance to personal success and prestige, particularly when obtained through strenuous striving against difficulties. Parental child-rearing strategies include expectations of high performances and responsibility coupled with a lack of emotional support needed for such achievements and for the development of an adequate sense of self-competence. These patterns of attachment, included in the vast group of "parental affectionless control" (Parker, 1983a), are frequently found in developmental experiences of depressive-prone individuals.

Eric (see p. 51) was sent to school almost a year and a half ahead of other children. His father, definitely a successful self-made man, was convinced from his own experience that an early struggle against difficulties would strengthen the boy's character and give him an advantage over others. A strong, life-toughened man, he considered any display of tenderness as dangerous for a good upbringing. The father's attitude toward Eric was fully in line with his beliefs. From the very first day of school, he firmly refused to consider Eric's younger age as a possible explanation of his mediocre performance. Instead, he ascribed it to the child's poor sense of responsibility and threatened him with severe measures, such as separation from the family by being sent to boarding school. Moreover, besides Eric's school performances (that improved only a little at a time and were, therefore, a major concern in Eric's childhood) the father's attitude embraced every possible aspect of Eric's life. For example, Eric was given a key to the house and instructed, from the first week of attendance, to go to school and come back alone.

3. *The inversion of the parent–child relationship, where the child is made responsible for the care of the parent* (Bowlby, 1980a). Frequently, one of the parents forces the child to take care of him/her by constantly accusing the child of being unlovable, incompetent, and inadequate. This is one more pattern of parental affectionless control in which the child is made to conform to strictly established standards by means of a steady, rejecting, and detached attitude, rather than by alternating inductions of responsibility and threats of desertion. In these cases the structuring of a sense of loss and personal loneliness is much more connected to a sense of self as unlovable and unworthy.

Lorna was a 36-year-old theater director who asked for psychotherapy because of intense depressive crises that accompanied her love relationships.

Her parents had separated when she was 3 years old and her father soon found another partner and left town. Lorna stayed with her fragile, emotionally unsteady mother who considered life an unsurmountable tragedy because of the selfishness of human beings. She would continually remind Lorna of the sacrifices she had made for her and accused her of being selfish for not paying her back with the affection and devotion she deserved. She also would tell Lorna that she was the only serious obstacle to a new love life. Lorna responded to the aggressive and punishing attitude with which her mother constantly requested care and assistance without openly rebelling because, little by little, she had become convinced that she was really responsible for her mother's unhappy situation. What was much less tolerable to her was the rejection she could sense in her mother's attitude. As far as she could recollect, she had always been the one to seek, in every possible occasion, contact with her mother, who, in turn, treated her with annoyance or open refusal. This was what caused, in early childhood, an unbearable sense of loneliness that she felt especially in school; faced with some problem, her friends could say, "I shall tell mother," and she realized that she could tell nobody.

In other circumstances, the inverted pattern of attachment seems to be a direct consequence of the death of one of the parents. In these cases, the greater request for care and assistance from the surviving parent seems to induce in the child a "caretaking" attitude. For example, some clients in our sample who had lost one parent clearly remembered their childhood decision to look after the other one.

IDENTITY DEVELOPMENT

The loss experience—whether scaffolded through real deaths or separations, or through parental patterns of affectionless control—seems to be at the core of the developing child's existing cognitive situation. The quality and intensity of the feelings that such experience can arouse deeply influence the child's unfolding patterns of self-perception and self-recognition.

Studies on bereavement and grief clearly support the notion of a reciprocal interdependence between the perception of loss and feelings of sadness and helplessness (Bowlby, 1961, 1973,

1980a; Parkes, 1972). This interconnection probably rests on the presence of genetically wired apprehensional schemata in which loss represents the more adaptive cognitive dimension for scaffolding important basic feelings (sadness and helplessness) into specific emotional schemata that may have great importance for survival and adaptation.

In the complex chain of processes defining the "unconditioned" relationship between loss and sadness, anger appears almost invariably as a relevant component. Because of opponent regulation processes that underly the dynamic equilibrium of any complex system, the emergence of anger represents the most effective and economical organismic device for preventing sadness and helplessness from becoming maladaptive. Consider, for example, the stages of despair, protest, and detachment that Bowlby (1973) describes as typical in children separated from their parents. In a systems approach, the entire process can be regarded as an ongoing, rhythmical and reciprocal regulation between opponent emotional polarities like helplessness (despair) and anger (protest) that reaches a sort of equilibrium only at the third stage, that is, detachment. Even if the family comes together again, the child is now reluctant to restore the emotional contact with the parent from whom he/she has been separated. It is as though striving to survive without a preferential attachment has become, in the meantime, an effective skill for coping with an adverse reality.

The centrality of the loss experience during early infancy will be reflected in the selective differentiation of opponent sets of prototypic emotional schemata as the bases underlying the subsequent emergence of a stable sense of self. At the end of preschool years, when these basic sets of emotional schemata have become sufficiently differentiated, amplified, and magnified to foster an initial rudimentary conceptualization, they can be ordered into a recursive loop oscillating between the opponent emotional polarities of sadness and anger.

In other words, the early ensembles of prototypical scenes about loss are formalized into a more stable nuclear scene (Tomkins, 1978) capable of providing the child with an equally stable sense of self. Because the continuous rehearsal of scenes concerning losses always brings a sense of one's being responsible for their occurring, the immediate sense of oneness that emerges is that of an unlovable person, uncapable of arousing in others positive feelings and attitudes, and incompetent in maintaining a secure relationship with an attachment figure. The consequential experience of loneliness also adds a sense of having to rely only on oneself in exploring the unknown surrounding world ("compulsive self-reliance"; Bowlby, 1977a).

The rhythmic oscillation between sadness and anger supplies a context of interdependent boundary constraints—with no single locus in ultimate control—within which the ongoing experiencing of self and world becomes increasingly articulated. Rapid oscillations between the two opponent boundaries are practically the rule in the first years of childhood—as though reality could be understood only through a series of alternating rejections and aggressive reactions. Later in childhood, because of the unfolding of cognitive growth, it becomes increasingly possible to actively seek intermediate emotional states, and thus to maintain a more acceptable proximity to others. The child generally stabilizes around a dynamic steady state by structuring an articulated pattern of decentralized controls. On the one hand, the exclusion of sensory inflow coming from critical domains (like rejections or failures) is even more selective and efficient; on the other hand, the repertoire of diversionary activities permits a certain degree of control over anger and opposing attitudes connected to anger, so as to further reduce the possibilities of rejection or failures.

As we can see, the developmental pathway that emerges from such patterns of decentralized control is one in which the continuous anticipation of losses and failures is experienced by the helpless child as the most effective way of reducing the intensity of disruptive emotions from losses and failures, perceived as certain and inevitable, that invariably occur. Thus, as has been observed in the first experimental models of animal learned helplessness (Seligman, 1974), the uncontrollability of traumatic experiential outcomes also seems to be a hallmark of human depressive developmental pathways. In an experimental study on attribution of success or failure following performances, Diener and Dweck (1980) found striking differences between helpless children and control groups. In addition, compared to mastery-oriented children, the helpless group underestimated the number of successes and overestimated the number of failures. Moreover, they did not regard successes as indicative of ability and did not expect them to continue. It was as though successes were less significant and predictive than failures.

ORGANIZATIONAL ASPECTS

The Adolescent Resolution

While, in the course of maturational stages, the developing subject builds a sense of his/her oneness by means of an immediate and concrete anticipation of losses and failures, with the adolescent reorganization this perceived oneness can produce a more articulated and inclusive way of ordering reality. The fundamental problem in the adolescent resolution of a depressive developmental pathway is to reach an equilibrium between two opponent, contradictory perceptions of self that are now available. On the one hand, the emergence of higher cognitive abilities promotes in the subject a sense of self as an actor that actively imposes its own order upon reality; while on the other, the perceived feeling of isolation and uncontrollability of experiential outcomes induces a sense of passiveness and helplessness that would nullify the ongoing attempt to elaborate a more active role.

In such a situation, the only condition that allows an equilibrium to be reached is for one to attribute the lack of control over ongoing experience to a perceived, stable internal trait—that is, to *decenter* uncontrollability from the immediate and negative appraisal of reality typical of childhood and *recenter* it on some negative perceived aspects of the self. In this way, the sense of passivity stemming from the perception of one's isolation and withdrawal can be actively matched with a parallel sense of activity deriving from the struggle against one's negativity in the effort to overcome it. The earlier sense of unlovableness and incompetence that in the course of the developmental pathway have become more and more differentiated in a compulsive self-reliant attitude toward reality undoubtedly exert a strong bias toward the structuring of this kind of self-blaming attitude.

In other words, the depressive attributional style described by the reformulated model of learned helplessness (Abramson, Seligman, & Teasdale, 1978; Seligman, Abramson, Semmel, & von Baeyer, 1979) in which, following failure, depressives tend to make internal attributions (effort, skill), whereas nondepressives tend to make external attributions (luck, task difficulty), appears to be the depressive's primary equilibration process from a systems perspective. Indeed, if a depressive adolescent reorganization assumed the opposite of an external, stable negative attribution, the individual would then perceive him/herself as helpless in an adverse, rejecting reality. A sense of self as an active agency could, in that case, be achieved only through the structuring of a paranoid, frightening nightmare of living in a hostile world. In fact, this could very well be one of the ways in which, starting from a depressive developmental pathway, a psychotic onset can occur during adolescence or early youth.

The Attitude toward Oneself and Reality

The commitment to oneself that emerges as a result of the structuring of a stable, negative internal attribution of losses and failures, is clearly expressed in reports that depressive-prone individuals give about their adolescence and youth. "If you work hard, have enough willpower to fight against your incompetence, and try to understand people's intentions and attitudes without ever getting angry or displaying opposing behaviors, you will be able to arouse attention and affection in others; and, eventually, you will succeed in avoiding loneliness and misery." With more or less these same words Eric and Lorna could have expressed, as adults, their adolescent intentions and commitment.

The developmental tacit, oscillative self-boundaries provide the apprehensional context within which the commitment to oneself can be progressively articulated into conscious models of self and the world (whose contents and structure vary according to the level of cognitive abstraction that the individual was able to attain). At times, the recursive oscillation between opponent emotional polarities makes a subject feel his/her perceived unlovableness as an intrinsic, unescapable characteristic of the self, toward which the only coherent attitude is a self-blaming one (sadness, helplessness). In other circumstances, it is perceived as something that can be strenuously fought against, and this attitude is accompanied by a feeling of competence and personal power in overcoming it (anger).

However, since the whole process consists in an oscillating regulation between opponent but simultaneously present emotional polarities, sadness and hopelessness are invariably more or less joined with anger. Therefore, especially when anger is poorly controlled—because of the quality and intensity of early losses— the individual is very likely to meet failures and rejections, and consequently, receives further confirmations of the crucial developmental experience concerning the uncontrollability of traumas. In relationships with others, the lack of control of anger leads to a characteristic interpersonal attitude in which outbursts of aggressive and provocative behaviors are intermingled with pleading and contact-seeking behaviors. Epidemiological and sociological literature shows that particularly severe cases of instability of early attachments often bring a high incidence of delinquency and antisocial personality (Rutter, 1972, 1979).

Moreover, inadequate control over anger also can have important repercussions on the subject's attitude toward him/herself. Besides producing uncontrollable social outcomes, a relevant portion of angry feelings can be scaffolded into a self-blaming, hopeless attitude toward oneself. This may explain the high rate in depressive-prone individuals of self-destructive behaviors such as suicidal ideations or attempts, and self-anesthetization with drugs or alcohol (Adam, 1982).[2]

As one can see, one of the most striking aspects of a depressive P.C.Org. consists of its marked tendency to produce in the cultural and social network a series of events, all of which are liable to be scaffolded in terms of losses and disappointments. Indeed, one might say that for the depressive-prone individual, the positive aspects of reality can be identified precisely by their inaccessibility; whereas the positive aspects of self can be identified by the continuous effort to try to adapt, at least in part, to this inaccessibility. In other words, an attitude toward oneself that organizes into patterns of compulsive self-reliance in order to reach an acceptable level of self-esteem necessarily requires for its articulation a steady confirmation of the experience of loneliness.

Consequently, the attitude toward reality is invariably centered on the perception of a gap between one's own and others' experiences that can be more or less insuperable according to the emotional oscillation in course—that is, whether others are perceived as indifferent or hostile and depending on the intensity and quality of anger aroused by specific loss experiences. The perception of this gap is usually maintained within the subject's stability range by an attitude toward affective relationships that is likely to produce a whole series of rejections or disappointments stemming from aloofness and apparent emotional detachment, "compulsive caregiving" (Bowlby, 1980a), or, as it happens most of the times, through the rhythmic oscillation of both. This kind of affectional style—that, as Brown suggests, could be phrased: "Those who give less have less to lose" (1982, p. 258)—clearly reflects the characteristic oscillative experiencing of loneliness of the depressive-prone individual. On the one side, loneliness is felt as a possible and dreadful lifelong destiny, while on the other, one's personal worth very likely depends on one's ability to face it.

SYSTEMIC COHERENCE

In a systemic perspective, the primacy of nuclear scenes concerning loss becomes evident as soon as we consider the equally central role that the experience of loneliness plays in the development and organization of a depressive P.C.Org. However, in childhood, isolation and withdrawal were immediate and concrete coping skills aimed at reducing the distressing perception of uncontrollability by anticipating failures and rejections; whereas during adolescence and youth they can be integrated into a more complex, compulsive self-reliant attitude that more abstractly aims at maintaining one's selected self-image within an acceptable level of self-esteem. Again, it is the organizational unity of the individual emotional domain that allows integrative shifts in the articulation of personal meaning processes within the same functional continuity.

The fact that reality itself becomes meaningful and increasingly ordered into personal experience only if continuously matched with the tacit experiencing of loss represents the pattern of organizational closure underlying the systemic coherence of a depressive P.C.Org. For example, the way in which Eric started to feel the emergence of a more defined sense of the future (as a consequence of the adolescence symmetry-breaking process in the perception of time) clearly reveals how the experiencing of loss becomes the basic, generative way of structuring new experiential domains.

At the end of childhood, Eric had gradually succeeded, through constant effort, to overcome the sense of impending failure and low self-competence that accompanied him from the time he began going to school. Therefore, in early adolescence, studying (the selected coping skill for striving against the impending loss represented by his father's threats of desertion) became his preferential strategy for achieving and maintaining an acceptable level of self-esteem and self-competence. At that same time, Eric started to actively avoid most social occasions with others his age; he preferred to stay in his father's library and look around or read through all the books that fascinated him. On one of those afternoons, when he was about 15 years old, he was enthusiastically contemplating the vastness of knowledge and suddenly had a distinct perception that all of his life would be spent acquiring that knowledge. Eric felt a flash of elation—one like he had never felt before, but for only an instant. The sense of fullness at once turned into deep despair and defeat. He was immediately aware that no matter how long he would live, the time would never be enough to embrace the immensity of knowledge that he now started to grasp. Eric's comment on this episode gave a fair idea of the centrality of his perception of loss in scaffolding the emergent projection into the future: "It was as though I felt old the first time I saw distinctly my future."

Besides generating new meaning domains, the perception of loss plays a fundamental role in assimilating experience inside already established experiential domains.

At 33 years of age, Lorna decided to end a love relationship that had lasted more than 5 years. This was the *first* time that she had ended a relationship (all her previous relationships were concluded by her partners). For quite some time before the separation, Lorna had felt doubtful and uncertain, expressing these feelings with constant and unpredictable oscillations between aggressive and provocative attitudes and contact-seeking behaviors. It was as though she were actually pushing her partner to make a decision. Faced with the submissiveness with which he accepted her attitudes, she finally made up her mind to leave him. Without experiencing the depressive reactions that usually accompanied her previous breakups, she felt as if she had gotten rid of a burden.

After some time, however, she started to have a recurring nightmare almost every night. The first few times that this occurred, she woke up in anguish and despair, having dreamed that her partner had insulted and laughed at her, saying that he had never been interested in her. He claimed that he had only pretended because he wanted to be close to her best friend, who was the woman he really loved and was now finally free to marry. In reporting the dream, Lorna admitted that this would have been a more "realistic" breakup for her and stated that her initiative had left her somehow "waiting," as though the relationship could not be considered really finished.

The continuous reproduction of the loss experience in depressive-prone individuals should not be regarded only as an abnormal and pathological feature, as if it merely consists of a sort of cumulative and passive reverberation of past schemata. On the contrary, it appears as an autonomous and creative knowing strategy whose generativeness and novelty production is based on the active construction of a sense of inaccessibility of reality. This explains why, when certain long-pursued goals are unexpectedly achieved, their positivity often abruptly changes into negativity. It is as if these goals too must necessarily turn out to be of little worth since they belong to a person of so little value. As Groucho Marx would have said, if a club accepted you as its member, then either the club has failed to recognize that there is something wrong with you (and thus proves that it is stupid), or else it has recognized it, but does not care (and has thus shown what kind of membership it has).

A knowing strategy of this kind has, of course, its own internal contradictions and discrepancies. If, in the course of intervening events, the sense of reality's inaccessibility goes beyond the individual's range of stability, the perception of uncontrollability of experiential outcomes prevails, activating a hopeless reaction that can in some cases take on the form of a true clinical depression.

On the other hand, as repeatedly pointed out, a system's internal contradictions and discrepancies are at the root of the generativity and directionality of its lifespan development. Therefore, due to the discontinuous emergence of these disequilibria and the subsequent attempts to assimilate them, a depressive P.C.Org. can reach, in the course of its temporal becoming, the levels of structural order and organized complexity compatible with its specific level of concreteness–abstractness dimension in experiencing loss.

THE DYNAMICS OF COGNITIVE DYSFUNCTION

In the last 10 years, cognitive theorists have outlined clinical models that accurately describe the behavioral and cognitive features usually observed in depressive disorders. A number of sources offer the reader an exhaustive and detailed description of the depressive symptomatology (Beck *et al.*, 1979; Guidano & Liotti, 1983; Shaw, 1979). In concluding this section, I will outline the systemic dynamics that underlie the onset of a clinical depression, as well as the interplay between the main processes involved.

Life events seemingly more capable of being scaffolded in terms of losses or disappointments, and therefore able to activate a disequilibrium in depressive-prone individuals, are schematized as follows by Brown and Harris (1978):

> (i) separation or threat of it . . .; (ii) an unpleasant revelation about someone close that forces a major reassessment of the person and the relationship . . .; (iii) a life-threatening illness to someone close; (iv) a major material loss or disappointment or the threat of it . . .; (v) an enforced change of residence or the threat of it; and finally (vi) a miscellaneous group of crises involving some elements of loss, such as being made redundant in a job held for some time, or obtaining a legal separation. (pp. 103–104)

A disequilibrium can activate a clinical depression when, as a result of tacit elaboration of ongoing experience, more integrated felt meanings concerning loss (that cannot be adequately decoded and assimilated in the conscious models of self and world) are made available. The basic dynamic is essentially as follows: The individual, though having the challenging possibility of articulating his/her personal and concrete experience of loss and loneliness toward a more abstract dimension (that would make them appear as problems occurring at the generalized level of mankind) nevertheless insists in regarding loss and loneliness as an uncontrollable and inescapable result of his/her perceived negativity.

Consider, for instance, Lorna's recurrent depressions whenever she experienced a sentimental disappointment. Although it was possible to start to suppose that the sense of loneliness was probably inherent to the human way of ordering interpersonal experience, Lorna—as her recurring nightmare shows—seemed to be able to consider it only as a direct consequence of her unlovableness and unworthiness. A more integrated experiencing of loneliness, in fact, seemed to now be available for Lorna, as her work of director and scriptwriter proved; her most recent works described loneliness as something strictly connected to the experience of love and intimacy itself. So, while her new emergent insights induced her to regard her supposed unlovableness from a different angle, she was firm in maintaining that it was her fault that the disappointment had occurred.

A disequilibrated depressive P.C.Org. exhibits, as a rule, patterns of cognitive dysfunction characterized by more or less intense helpless reactions.

However, since hopelessness is a complex emotion common in every human being because of its importance for survival and adaptation, it becomes necessary to make a clinical distinction between the typical helplessness exhibited by a depressive-prone individual and that which can be recognized as a common response to adversity in any P.C.Org. While in the latter case, hopelessness is always specifically limited to the experiential domain that elicited it, in a depressive P.C.Org. the hopeless reaction generalizes to the point of being felt as the hopelessness of one's life as a whole (Brown, 1982).

The generalized helpless reaction is usually matched by a marked decrease in the rate of activity, which can sometimes be reduced to a state of inertia and total immobility. Reduced interests and activity are to be considered a direct expression, at the cognitive–behavioral level, of the actual experienced helplessness and, therefore, vary accordingly. The way of coping with ongoing experience is still permeated by the individual's attitude toward reality; that is, strenuous striving is needed in order to confront the toughness of life. But now the conclusions are reversed. Since one is helpless in the face of one's wicked fate (which one deserves) the most logical and economical thing to do is to remain passive, so at least one will spare effort.

The discrepancy between one's challenging feelings about loss and one's selected conscious models of self and world is generally marked by an interplay between simultaneous and competing processes that can be outlined as follows.

1. At the conscious explicit level, the subject's attempts to maintain the usual self-image is mainly expressed through the elaboration of theories supporting a negative view of the self, the world, and the future. These negative views generally apply to the individual's personal domain, that is, to those aspects of self and world that were meaningful and valued before the onset of depression. This is the well-known *cognitive triad of depression*, originally described by Beck (1967) and considered a central feature by current cognitive models of clinical depression (Beck, 1976; Guidano & Liotti, 1983; Shaw, 1979; Shaw & Dobson, 1981).

This characteristic thematic content of depressive cognition—that in the more serious cases comes with more or less elaborated beliefs of suffering from a mental disease—can be considered to be at the core of diversionary activities with which the subject directs his/her attention from further processing challenging feelings by focusing on his/her perceived misery.

2. At the tacit level, the activation of challenging feelings about loss, with the impossibility of a more adequate and comprehensive cognitive scaffolding, will tend to manifest itself through emotional outbursts in which helplessness and anger are continuously intermingled. Moreover, because of the low cognitive control, the motor pattern that accompanies the oscillating interplay between helplessness and anger will tend to be directly realized by a continuous alternation of inertia and self-destructive behaviors.

A depressive cognitive dysfunction tends to fade away spontaneously with the passing of time, as clinical observation has long since shown. Even individuals who have not reached an acceptable integration of challenging feelings usually find that relative control can be regained over most of their ongoing events as soon as the stressful life event passes. In such instances, the depressive P.C.Org. readjusts itself into its more adaptive form. These cases, however, stand on a very narrow-margin equilibrium that, consequently is much more likely to become unstable whenever it is confronted with even minimal losses or disappointments.

NOTES

1. It is common knowledge that the nosological status of depression is rather controversial. To avoid as much as possible the risk of mixing conditions that could perhaps be heterogeneous, data pertaining to clients has been limited to those who would have been diagnosed as neurotic, psychogenic, and reactive depressives by most psychiatrists.

2. Interesting experimental data from research on endorphins suggest the existence of an interdependence between the brain opiate system and the development of social attachments. Support for such interdependence is provided by the fact that separation distress may be paralleled by an endogenous activity *reduction* in the brain opiate system and that the *activation* of the brain opiate system (via administration of small amounts of morphine) has a specific effect in the relief of the separation distress (Panksepp, Herman, Conner, Bishop, & Scott, 1978). Obviously, future developments in this kind of research could supply precious information about the complex processes that govern the loss–separation dimension, and about the role that these processes play in the facilitation of self-destructive and self-anesthetizing behaviors observed in depressive P.C.Orgs.

CHAPTER EIGHT

THE AGORAPHOBIC COGNITIVE ORGANIZATION

Fear is sharp-sighted, and can see things under ground, and much more in the skies. —Cervantes

The organizational unity of a phobic-prone individual's emotional domain is based on a dynamic steady equilibrium between two opponent emotional polarities: (1) the need for protection from a perceived dangerous world, and (2) the need for freedom and independence in the same world. The most outstanding feature of this kind of organizational pattern is a marked tendency to respond in terms of fear and anxiety (and a more or less intense reduction of autonomous behavior) to any alteration in the balance of affectional bonds that may be scaffolded by the individual in terms of loss of protection and/or loss of freedom and independence (Guidano, in press; Guidano & Liotti, 1983, 1985).

Using the same format employed in the previous chapter, the developmental and organizational processes underlying the systemic coherence of an agoraphobic P.C.Org. will be illustrated.[1]

DYSFUNCTIONAL PATTERNS OF ATTACHMENT

The central core of the developmental pathway of an agoraphobic P.C.Org. consists of a class of maturational experiences all of which, despite their diversity, are characterized by an *indirect* interference or limitation of the child's autonomous exploratory behavior.

In a large majority of cases, this interference results from patterns of anxious attachment established by parents lacking emotional warmth, who nevertheless indirectly succeed in keeping a close bond with their children by either frightening them with descriptions of an outside world full of dangers, or by restraining them with threats of desertion (Arrindell, Emmelkamp, Monsma, & Brilman, 1983; Bowlby, 1969, 1973, 1983; Parker, 1979, 1983b).

For the sake of conciseness, the vast variety of these dysfunctional patterns of attachment that limit the child's exploratory behavior can be subsumed under two large categories that can also occur in combination with each other.

1. *Limitation of the child's exploratory behavior by an overprotective parent behavior.* A typical feature of this group of attachment patterns involves the parent portraying the world as a threatening and dangerous place, while at the same time impressing upon the child that he/she is weak and particularly vulnerable to these perils.

While such parenting behavior is usually an expression of the parents' intolerance of the child's normal separation initiatives, they invariably justify the restrictions imposed on the child's freedom as not depending on their own wishes. For example, even in the frequent cases of phobic-prone parents who actively retain the child with them because of their fear of being home alone, it is never explicitly stated that they prefer to have their children nearby for their own pleasure or company. On the contrary, reasons given by parents for limiting autonomy always concern an alleged weakness of the child of either a physical nature (e.g., "you are frail") or of an emotional nature (e.g., "you don't know how to control yourself in front of other people"). As a matter of fact, it is the parents' overprotecting attitude that makes the child not only perceive such weakness as real, but to also accept it and take it for granted.

Ever since she could remember, Shirley (see p. 74) always had the impression that she was "feeble" and, therefore, that she had to be more careful about her health than other girls. When she was born, her father, a renowned doctor, was already a middle-aged man. Although he was brusque and undemonstrative, from the outset he established a preferential relationship with her. However, almost the only way in which her father expressed his attachment was by a physical overprotection that often had tragicomic overtones. For example, when Shirley and other girls in her class fell ill with measles, her father, fearing the possibility of meningitis, was so scrupulous and lengthy in treating her that she was kept home for 6 months and missed the whole school year. Even the slightest cold or flu always required long convalescences and absences from school in order to be sure that any possible aftereffect or relapse had been prevented. Restrictions in games with schoolmates, outings, trips, and so on always followed the same rules, that is, prevent diseases or accidents by limiting physical strain, sweats, and so on.

The different life Shirley felt she led compared to her friends was, however, not experienced as isolation, nor did it make her feel sad. She felt that her father, despite his gruff and apparently distant manner, was very attached to her, perhaps because of that very "feebleness" that, according to a family rumor, she might have acquired from her mother. That was why Shirley, rather than upsetting her father, always agreed to stay home with him. So, even when (soon after puberty) her father started to warn her about the possible physical and psychological disturbances that might result from intimate relationships, Shirley took it for granted that her well-known feebleness could now appear in the form of emotional frailty.

2. *Limitation of the child's exploratory behavior through a rejecting parental attitude.* The significant element in this category is the fact that parents are not apt to be perceived by the child as a safe base, and this makes him/her feel insecure when outside the home. In other words, children refrain from autonomously exploring the environment for fear of losing their parents if they get too far from them.

A rather common situation occurs when an uneffusive parent, lacking emotional warmth, tries to obtain positive attention from the child by threatening to leave the family, attempting suicide, or complaining of suffering from an incurable disease that will soon result in death. Another frequent situation is that of a parent who suffers from chronic anxiety due to loneliness, and blames the child for an imminent severe sickness that might seize him/ her when alone and helpless. This is basically another case of inversion of the parent/child relationship in which the control of the child's behavior is obtained by forcing him/her to take care of the parent.

Since early childhood, Albert (see p. 118) reported having been afraid of losing his parents—especially his mother, since his father, who was away all the time, was merely a figure whose existence he knew about. His mother was a rigid, undemonstrative woman, crushed under the burden of an unsatisfactory marriage and a catastrophic financial situation, who expressed her unhappiness by claiming that she was sick and merely waiting to be liberated by death. At times she abandoned herself to melodramatic scenes; she would take Albert in her arms and say tearfully: "My poor little darling, what will you do when I am gone?"

Going to kindergarten was agony for Albert, he always feared that something could happen to his mother while he was away. He especially remembered having been terrified on a couple of occasions when his mother had not come to fetch him; both times he had felt sure she was dead. He felt reassured only when he began elementary school. The school building was right next to his home and from where he sat, he could see the windows of his apartment and make sure his mother was there, moving about the house.

IDENTITY DEVELOPMENT

Therefore, at the center of the developing child's existing situation is the limitation of his/her exploratory behavior experienced as something naturally connected to the maintenance of an adaptive proximity to attachment figures.

The indirectness of such limitation has important consequences. It prevents children from experiencing the emotional distress from the perceived limitation as something coming directly from parental coercion. If this were the case, the structuring of opposing or openly rebellious attitudes to parents' educational policies would be much more likely. Conversely, the emotional distress is experienced as part of a more complex situation that is perceived as the effect of being lovingly protected from imaginary dangers, and/ or as something absolutely necessary for their presumed condition of having to face the threat of desertion and loneliness (Guidano & Liotti, 1983, 1985).

In this state of affairs, the most outstanding effect concerns the relationship between attachment and exploration, that is, between two classes of interdependent and genetically rooted behaviors. The separation initiatives that the child shows at the beginning of exploratory behavior, in fact, do not in any way indicate the end of attachment, nor does separation represent the opposite polarity to attachment. On the contrary, attachment and separation should be regarded as "interplay classes of behaviors which develop side by side and coexist throughout the life of an individual" (Rheingold & Eckerman, 1970, p. 79).

A healthy and balanced cognitive–emotional development, therefore, results from the ongoing rhythmical and reciprocal regulation between these two classes of interdependent behaviors. While attachment is the safe base that allows the activation of a confident exploratory behavior capable of autonomously assimilating the novelties presented by the environment, the progressive unfolding of exploratory behavior influences the further articulation and the quality of attachment itself. The emergence of conceptual perspective taking and related cognitive skills allows children to communicate to other people who are significant to them the experiences that they have had during their own exploration. In this way, normal separation development permits relational structures of attachment to develop further so that attachment will include not only patterns of physical contact, but also patterns for communicating one' opinions and emotions.

In the developing phobic-prone child on the other hand, *attachment and separation processes ultimately acquire an antithetical correlation* to each other. Therefore, their interdependence can be expressed only through a rhythmical and opponent regulation between mutually antagonistic polarities—as if one should necessarily exclude the other. As a result, from the earliest stages of development, the subject will carry out a selective differentiation of opponent sets of prototypical emotional schemata as the basis underlying the subsequent emergence of a stable sense of self.

On the one side, the rehearsal of scenes concerning the limitation of inborn tendencies toward autonomous environmental exploration is reflected in the need for freedom and independence. This, however, necessarily implies the likely frightening experiences of loneliness and lack of protection from dangerous novelties coupled with alleged personal weakness and low self-competence. In contrast, the perception of the external world as a perilous threatening place is reflected in a need for protection by close physical proximity to attachment figures. This inevitably implies a likely repetition of the distressing experience of constriction and limitation.

When these prototypical emotional schemata are formalized into a more ordered nuclear scene at the end of preschool years, a stable self-recursive loop unfolds that oscillates between antithetical emotional polarities and supplies the decoding context underlying the child's contradictory experiencing of self. Although the continuous safety and attention provided by overprotective parents have allowed the child to elaborate a sense of self as a lovable and valuable person, the perceived restriction of independence matched with memories of frightening experiences in facing environmental novelties have allowed the elaboration of a sense of self as a weak and incompetent person.

However, due to the unfolding of cognitive growth, the child is now able to maintain within tolerable limits the discrepant perception of self by actively seeking the intermediate states within his/her oscillative boundary constraints represented by the frightening experiences of loneliness and constriction. This dynamic steady state is usually obtained through the structuring of specific patterns of decentralized control—that is, by (1) progressively excluding all sensory inflow capable of activating needs of freedom and independence, and (2) by structuring a repertoire of somatic and visceral complaints that act as diversionary activities for maintaining proximity to protective figures without having to reduce one's perceived self-esteem.

It should be evident that this process leads to the differentiation of a developmental pathway capable of avoiding the frightening experiences connected to loneliness and constriction by means of an active self-control directed toward excluding one's challenging feelings and emotional experiences. Because the possibility of an adequate emotional differentiation is further reduced by the lack of emotional warmth and tenderness typical of family patterns of attachment (in which affection is mainly expressed with physical overprotection) and by the limited chances to explore and autonomously discover new emotional domains, one can readily understand how the conscious emotional range of the phobic-prone adolescent is quite undifferentiated and restricted.

In particular, during the course of development, many ensembles of emotional schemata have been insufficiently transformed into semantic cognitive content. Consequently, the information contained in feelings primarily remains stored, represented, and retrieved through other channels—that is, perception, imagery–memory mechanism, and motor patterns. The activation of these emotional schemata is, therefore, likely to be expressed by muscular–visceral reactions paralleled by the emergence of somewhat undecodable feelings and images in the stream of consciousness. This obviously further stabilizes the "object-bound" attitude of seeking a proper self-control on one's sense of fragility and inadequacy through the achievement of an adequate, secure proximity to protective figures. Fear, activated by the constant oscillation between the need for freedom and the need for protection, is undoubtedly the most structured and easily recognizable feeling within this emotional range.

As a final consideration, I would like to point out that the principle domains of phobic personal meaning processes—that is, needs for freedom, protection, and self-control—are mainly based on the parents' apprehension of the world and the child's imagination of dangers and isolation, rather than on events that have actually occurred. Generally, the only developmental stressful experience that really takes place involves the limitation of one's inborn tendency to explore the environment. But this pertains to one's tacit realm and can hardly be verbalized, even after the emergence of abstract–formal thought processes. As previously noted about the depressive cognitive organization, actual stressful experiences of isolation and loneliness during childhood lead to different developmental pathways, ones in which fear is not so strongly implied.

ORGANIZATIONAL ASPECTS

The Adolescent Resolution

With the emergence of higher cognitive abilities, the phobic-prone individual must develop a more stable equilibration of the discrepant aspects that underlie his/her perceived oneness. In this process it is possible for the sense of self as a controlling agency, elaborated in childhood, to be transformed into a more articulated and active actor's sense of self. In order for this to occur though, one must reorganize one's parallel perceived sense of weakness and inadequacy that stems from the limits attributed to the self in facing novel and unfamiliar environments.

As a rule, the most readily available solution involves attributing one's need for protection to a stable and negative external cause, that is, toward an "objectively" dangerous and coercive reality. In contrast to what usually happens in the depressive developmental pathway, the phobic adolescent's resolution involves *decentering* the experienced limitation of one's freedom of action from the immediate perception of one's supposed weakness, more typical of childhood, and *recentering* it on some negative perceived aspect of reality.[2]

In other words, phobic-prone adolescents identify their "real self" with the need for freedom and commit themselves to a self-image that excludes certain aspects (weakness, emotionality, fear of loneliness, etc.) that would make them depend on other people—just like they depended on their parents in the past. This inevitably implies the structuring of increasingly sophisticated controlling skills for excluding a whole range of critical feelings and emotions that might challenge the selected self-image. Thus, the commitment to oneself as a controlling agent progressively influences the development of a defined sense of personal identity; one in which emotionality and effusive behaviors are identified with personal weaknesses and, consequently, excluded from one's conscious emotional range. Self-competence is therefore based on the strict identification of personal emotions with controllable emotions, while self-esteem and self-worthiness tend to be strictly equated to self-control.

The Attitude toward Oneself and Reality

With this kind of commitment to him/herself, a phobic-prone individual generally succeeds in achieving a steady and dynamic equilibrium between the opponent needs for protection and freedom, while at the same time allowing him/herself to maintain an acceptable level of self-esteem and self-competence.

The recursive oscillation between antithetical emotional polarities (need for protection vs. need for freedom) allows one's sense of being a controlling agent to be perceived either as self-reliance—if based upon confirmation of one's ability to find in every possible new circumstance other available protective figures (need for protection)—or as autonomy and independence—if based upon confirmation of one's ability to control interpersonal relationships able to provide an adequate sense of protection (need for freedom). On the other hand, a recursivity of this kind implies a tendency to react with a unique emotional intensity to specific variations of one's affectional balance. In particular, this may occur in reaction to threats of detachment (however imaginary) from protective figures, and conversely, to any increase of emotional involvement in an ongoing affective relationship that can be perceived as a limitation of one's freedom of action. Inside this oscillative process, phobic-prone individuals are able to maintain their stable ongoing felt identity through an external attributive attitude. As a consequence, they experience such emotions not so much as the outcome of their own personal affectional style, but rather as con- firmations of the existence of a dangerous and coercive reality.

The phobic attitude toward oneself is exemplified in the way the individual attempts to overcontrol feelings and emotions. This overcontrol is brought about in the first place by the tendency to assume a sort of "object-bound" attitude toward oneself in which feelings and emotions are regarded as external to the self. Controlling procedures are therefore based on an almost automatic prevention or avoidance of emotions, rather than on their understanding in terms of personal meaning (Guidano & Liotti, 1983, 1985). The poor differentiation of the individual's range of decodable emotions that occurred in the course of development probably adds to a further stabilization of the overcontrolling object-bound attitude. In fact, it is known that whenever there are difficulties in using appropriate cognitive labels for decoding one's ongoing emotional experiences, the latter are generally experienced as alien and more or less unpleasant (Bowlby, 1979; Marshall & Zimbardo, 1979; Maslach, 1979).

Finally, in dealing with emotions connected to variations in the affectional balance, the overcontrolling attitude is intensified to the point of making the individual "blind" to certain personal emotional experiences.[3] This selective exclusion of challenging data is mainly brought about by what Bowlby (1980a) would call the cognitive disconnection of one's emotional response from the interpersonal situation that elicited it. When the disconnection is complete, the response appears totally unintelligible in terms of one's reactions to threats of loneliness or constriction and can be better explained by invoking causes external to the self, like somatic or psychological complaints.

The phobic attitude toward reality is also characterized by the way in which the individual manages to obtain a secure proximity to protective figures while at the same time avoiding the frightening experience of a limitation of one's freedom of action. The overcontrolling attitude toward significant others is effected through a selective attention to formal and metacommunicative features (contextual and nonverbal cues) of ongoing interactions rather than to content of such interactions. Thus, it becomes possible to maintain a stable "one-up" role through continuous redefinitions of the formal aspects of the relationship and to manipulate it according to one's need for protection or control.

Finally, the overcontrolling attitude tends to be intensified in intimate relationships, because they can arouse the most intense and involved emotions. The phobic-prone individual's affectional style is characterized by the constant attempt to have a reference figure at his/her disposal, while at the same time being careful to avoid feeling dependent and limited in one's freedom of movement. Men, for example, often exhibit brilliant, outgoing, and assertive social behavior and have many superficial affairs charged predominantly with sexual interest, so as to avoid as much as possible any stable emotional commitment. Women, on the other hand, have a marked tendency toward orgasmic dysfunction, revealing most of the time an almost deliberate attempt to maintain control in the relationship with their sexual partner. Because they are so sensitive to the formal aspects of the relationship, this difficulty can often be overcome if they take the upper position during intercourse; only feeling constricted or oppressed when the reverse position is assumed.

SYSTEMIC COHERENCE

The overcontrolling attitude toward oneself and reality that progressively emerges after the adolescent resolution, is, therefore, the basic strategy for the attainment of a steady and dynamic equilibrium between the opposite and conflicting needs for freedom and protection. A balance of this kind, of course, has its own internal contradictions and incongruities.

The most outstanding is undoubtedly the discrepancy between the individual's tendency to seek steady affective relationships that are capable of supplying adequate protection, and his/her inability to master the existential and emotional aspects pertaining to the human affective domain. In fact, having to mostly concentrate on the formal aspects of human relationships and on the immediate and concrete aspects of interpersonal and intrapersonal control, the phobic-prone individual is incapable of developing an adequate knowledge of all the shades and complexities implied in the formation, maintenance, and breaking of affectional bonds. Moreover, in order to avoid an expression of personal weakness, he/she must exclude from the conscious emotional range any emotion that reveals a dependence upon others. Thus, phobic-prone individuals find it difficult to recognize as their own the emerging emotional involvement toward significant others. Therefore, making new affective bonds, breaking old ones, or perceiving growing loneliness or constriction in an ongoing significant relationship can easily produce feelings and emotional experiences whose control would require the elaboration of more complex explanations than those allowed by the individual's controlling attitude.

However, it is through the integration of disequilibria produced by the emergence of these challenging data that a phobic P.C.Org. can undergo a progressive widening of the conscious range of personal emotions and consequently have the possibility of reaching more integrated and comprehensive balances between its central, antithetical needs. The fact that reality itself becomes meaningful and increasingly ordered into personal experience only if continuously matched with the recursive oscillation between the need for freedom and the need for protection therefore represents the pattern of organizational closure underlying the systemic coherence of a phobic P.C.Org. For instance, the way in which Shirley (see pp. 74, 140), at age 24, felt and recognized the emotional involvement that bound her to her boyfriend, clearly illustrates how an unpleasant increase of the need for protection can be a generative way of structuring new experiential domains in one's emotional life.

The first frightening experiences of being courted by boys confirmed in Shirley the idea that in order to be a strong, efficient, and self-controlled woman, she had to avoid any stable emotional commitment. She had acquired a brilliant, assertive, and seductive attitude, and was now able to manage several affairs simultaneously. In this way she could prevent any one of them from becoming more exclusive. She kept control of her emotional involvement by not surrendering herself completely during intercourse and by immediately concentrating on another affair as soon as the current one became, in spite of herself, more involving. As a result, in recent years her love life had become somewhat agitated, to the point that several times she was tempted to go back to a quieter, more orderly, life.

This was the explanation she gave to herself when she decided to establish a steady relationship with the man who would eventually become her husband. His complete submissiveness seemed to guarantee that she would be able to control all aspects of the relationship. Although this engagement appeared to be a long-lasting one, Shirley reassured herself by firmly believing that this was a free relationship and that she did *not* love him. After some time, however, she began to gradually end all her other affairs. She explained this by convincing herself that, because she felt reassured by the steady but not involved relationship, she could now dedicate more time to her work and career (which she thought she had previously neglected). She had thus reached an equilibrium that involved preventing herself (by overcontrolling her emotions) from becoming aware of the involvement that she was actually tacitly establishing with her future husband.

This narrow-margin equilibrium became unstable as soon as Shirley experienced her first orgasm with him. She immediately decided to spend a weekend with an office colleague who had been pressuring her to have an affair. However, while packing her suitcase, she felt an odd physical breakdown coming over her, matched by a pervading sense of being unable to go or to do anything else without her boyfriend near her, protecting her. It was mostly because of this experience (which Shirley carefully avoided reporting to her mate) that she agreed to revise the attribution of "non importance" to this relationship, and began to make explicit marriage plans.

In considering once more the circumstance in which Albert (see p. 118) had his first panic attack, it can be noticed in this case also that the surfacing of an unexpected feeling of constriction (which signaled a surging awareness of the monotony and dullness of his marital relationship) should have led him to revise his beliefs about the nature of affectional bonds to conclude that they were more important to him than he had thought. The fact that Albert came to this conclusion after cognitive psychotherapy in no way diminishes the consideration that this emergence of uncontrollable feelings of constriction and/or loneliness is the underlying basis for the generativity and directionality of a phobic lifespan development. In fact, apart from the technical mode in which they are carried out, the attempts to assimilate challenging pressures during the course of his/her life enable a phobic-prone individual to reach a greater integration of self-awareness—compatible with his/her own particular level on the concreteness–abstractness dimension—in experiencing the antinomy between the need for freedom and the need for protection.

THE DYNAMICS OF COGNITIVE DYSFUNCTION

Life events capable of activating challenging pressures that may precipitate the onset of a clear-cut agoraphobic picture can be subsumed into two large groups.

1. Real or imaginary situations apt to be scaffolded in terms of loss of protection that can consequently activate intense fears of impending loneliness.

Rather than a real or threatened separation, the individual sometimes experiences a general increase in the need for freedom and independence due to maturational advancement. Following adolescent maturation, for instance, one can feel stronger thrusts toward a greater emotional distancing from parents and the formation of new affectional bonds. Shirley's case (see p. 74) is a typical example of an onset of this kind during adolescence. Moreover, a number of investigators have suggested a direct transition from school phobia to agoraphobia (Berg, Butler, & Hall, 1976; Berg, Marks, McGuire, & Lipsedge, 1974). In fact, apart from adolescence, any life period in which the person must face greater independence can be regarded as a stage of special vulnerability for the phobic-prone individual (Weiss, 1964). Such periods may occur during youth when the anticipation of forthcoming work means becoming independent from parents, or during adulthood when the disposition toward more money and leisure promotes the need for greater freedom and autonomy.

In other situations, fear of loneliness begins soon after the threatened or actual loss of a significant person. Generally, it involves the death of one of the parents or abandonment (or the threat of it) by a husband, wife, or significant partner.

2. Change in the balance of an ongoing significant affective relationship apt to be scaffolded in terms of loss of freedom and independence, and therefore arousing intense, uncontrollable feelings of constriction.

In some cases, changes experienced by the individual seem to coincide directly with the formation of an affectional bond itself because initial panic attacks occur in close correlation with marriage, often during the honeymoon (Liotti & Guidano, 1976). In other circumstances, a marital crisis makes the individual aware of a sense of constriction because, for several reasons, he/she now perceives the desired or imagined separation as impossible. Albert's case in Chapter 6 can be included in this group. Finally, other situations concern modifications of the relationship not experienced as marital crises. The most typical example is the birth of a child, often unexpected, and the consequent redistribution of family tasks between husband and wife that result in a perceived loss of independence for one of the two.

A disequilibrated agoraphobic P.C.Org. generally exhibits a variety of specific cognitive and behavioral disorders that has been amply described in the literature (Beck, 1976; Coleman, 1981; Emmelkamp, 1982; Guidano & Liotti, 1983, 1985; Marks, 1969; Mathews, Gelder, & Johnston, 1981). Consistent with the perspective taken up to this point, an outline of the systemic dynamics of the agoraphobic disorder will be presented.

The discrepancy between the emergent, intense feelings of loneliness and/or constriction and the conscious accepted image of self as a controlling agent generally results in an interplay between simultaneous and competing processes. These can be briefly outlined as follows.

1. At the conscious level, the individual cannot help experiencing the presence of unbearable feelings such as *fear of losing control*. The images and internal dialogues that refer to the possibility of losing control vary in intensity and content from case to case. Most of the time they take the form of images related to loss of consciousness due of fainting or heart attacks, to sequences showing an impending madness, or to the total inability to face a physical ill-being. Without a doubt the fear of losing control in situations that can activate feelings of constriction and/or loneliness is the hallmark of an agoraphobic cognitive dysfunction.

As a rule, this fear is connected to representations concerning external danger and centered on the idea that strangers (i.e., nonfamiliar persons) can be hostile and dangerous. As an inevitable result, the subject's representations are centered on disapproval, ridicule, criticism, or even physical aggression from unknown bystanders. In any case, motor autonomy is considerably reduced and the person actively seeks the company of a trustworthy familiar person both while staying at home and during his/her everyday movements.

The subject's attempt to maintain his/her established self-image is usually expressed with the elaboration of theories that prove the alien nature of the perceived discrepancy. A proliferation of *disease theories* then takes place to explain a supposed mysterious weakness or fragility of the body or mind. This vague feeling of personal weakness though, should merely be regarded as an almost tautological consequence of the individual's external causal attribution. In the face of a reality conceived as unsupported and coercive, one cannot help perceiving oneself as somehow weak and limited.

However, the perception of this alleged weakness does not reduce the agoraphobic's self-esteem. They consider themselves weak, but not unlovable; and physically inferior because of a disease, not because of incompetence. In other words, by adding the connotation of illness to their self-image, they succeed in having a consistent explanation for their distressing feelings without having to modify their accustomed level of self-esteem.

The characteristic thematic contents of agoraphobic cognitions (perceived fear of losing control and physical danger) are at the core of the various diversionary activities through which these individuals prevent themselves from becoming fully aware of their emotional life. In fact, as shown by common clinical observation, the bound attitude toward the spouse prevents the individual from taking seriously the images of liberation and escape from marriage that usually come with his/her feelings of loneliness and constriction (see the case of Albert, p. 118). Wolpe (1976), for instance, has stated that one of the most common ways of developing a fear of being alone originates from the presence of recurring fantasies of liberation from an unsatisfactory marriage. These fantasies remain unfullfilled precisely because they evoke great fear (p. 161).

2. At the tacit level, the activation of challenging feelings that cannot be more adequately and comprehensively scaffolded will tend to manifest itself through emotional outbursts in which fear of loneliness and constriction are always intermingled with the fear of losing control. Furthermore, since reality is tacitly and immediately experienced as coercive and/or unsupported (due to an external causal attribution that is now completely automatic) the behavior and autonomic activation that accompany the arousal of critical feelings will tend to be directly realized in the two previously described situations: (a) loneliness, marked by the absence of a trustworthy companion in the immediate surroundings (e.g., being alone at home, in a public place, and so on); (b) constriction, that is, situations felt as limiting one's freedom of movement (i.e., traffic jams, elevators, crowded places, buses or subways from which one cannot get out at one's will, etc.).

Over time, the trend of an agoraphobic cognitive dysfunction, though extremely variable, shows a certain tendency to maintain and stabilize itself (unlike depressive disorders). In a certain number of cases, however, a natural readjustment is possible. This primarily occurs in those favorable situations where the subject achieves an acceptable integration of the disequilibrium accompanied by a progressive shift in self-awareness, or where the perceived threat of impending loneliness or constriction was caused by either temporary or exceptional circumstances, and consequently vanishes as soon as the latter cease to exist.

In other situations, the phobic behavior apparently tends to become stabilized because it allows the individual to recover at least part of his/her overcontrolling attitude in the relationship and prevents the partner from threatening desertion or demanding greater autonomy or power. To quote an example, Liotti and Guidano (1976) reported a typical pattern of interpersonal behavior between some male agoraphobics and their wives. When agoraphobia emerged in these relationships, a sort of stable and paradoxical balance regarding dominance and submission developed. The wife appeared to be the "one-up" in the relationship because she was protecting and accompanying her troubled husband just as one might assist a sick or childish person. But it was the husband who actually had control of the couple's activities and dominated his wife by deciding what could be done and what could not. This depended to a large extent on whether he would be likely to have an anxiety attack.

NOTES

1. The nosographic perspective underlying the present discussion considers the multiform and diversified aspects of anxiety and phobic disorders to be the expression of a unitary syndrome, because they are produced by similar etiologic and pathogenic mechanisms. Therefore, the term "agoraphobia" is applied to all those cases presenting the *fear of facing certain situations alone*, although in many instances some fears seem to assume greater intensity or significance than the fear of loneliness (see Guidano & Liotti, 1983).

2. Quite obviously, a stable external causal attribution of this kind, if combined with cognitive processes that are poorly developed in relation to abstracting ability and integration, can give rise to attitudes and behaviors commonly labeled "psychotic." In clinical practice, for example, it is not uncommon to find agoraphobics who carry guns in their cars or on their person, in order to be able to face the hostility and possible physical violence that they attribute to strangers.

3. Hamlyn (1977), among others, has described a pattern of attitude toward oneself that he calls "blindness to oneself." This is characterized by a "refusal" to commit oneself to the achievement of an integrated level of self-awareness because of an overriding attention to the actual environment.

CHAPTER NINE

THE EATING DISORDERS
COGNITIVE ORGANIZATION

I think I like myself, but I'm not so sure I have good taste. —Altan[1]

The oneness of personal meaning processes in eating disorder-prone individuals stems from a blurred perceived sense of the self and organizes itself around deep boundaries that oscillate between an absolute need for significant others' approval and the fear of being intruded upon or disconfirmed by significant others. The relevant feature of this kind of organizational pattern is a marked tendency to alter the body image through dysfunctional eating patterns (anorexia, obesity, bulimia, binge–purge syndrome, thin–fat people's syndrome, etc.). These patterns emerge in response to any perceived disequilibrium between the previously mentioned opponent emotional polarities (Bruch, 1973, 1978, 1980; Guidano, in press; Guidano & Liotti, 1983; Minuchin, Rosman, & Baker, 1978; Selvini-Palazzoli, 1978).

INVARIANT ASPECTS OF DYSFUNCTIONAL
PATTERNS OF ATTACHMENT

So variegated a range of clinical disorders may originate from a number of possible dysfunctional patterns of attachment. For a clearer exposition, therefore, the invariant aspects that underlie the variability of the surface features that these patterns can assume will be directly analyzed.

The most remarkable element of the developmental pathway of an eating disorder P.C.Org. consists of the fact that these invariant aspects, in combining with each other, produce a specific discrepant experience in the child's unfolding sense of self. On the one hand, because of an ambiguous, undefined attachment style, the child can achieve a stable self-perception only through an *enmeshed relationship with an attachment figure.* But on the other, during childhood or adolescence the individual invariably experiences *disappointment with the same attachment figure.* This once again makes the achievement of a stable sense of self problematic.

Once this common feature is understood, it is possible, through a developmental analysis, to reconstruct the specific patterns that such discrepant experience has assumed.

Enmeshed Patterns of Attachment

The typical family environment of most eating disorder-prone individuals is characterized by disguised ambiguous, and contradictory communication.

Parents are usually extremely attentive to formal aspects of life—especially social appearances. Their primary purpose is to provide an image of a perfectly happy marriage by avoiding any outward expression of defined emotions or opinions that would hint at the existence of problems and reciprocal unsatisfactions. Therefore, there is a strong tendency to conceal any personal difficulty or contradiction, whether pertaining to their present interaction with the world or to their past. Similarly, they tend to offer an image of themselves as parents entirely dedicated to the well-being and upbringing of their children. Their parenting behavior, however, is directed more toward obtaining for themselves a confirmation of that image than at fulfilling their children's concrete need for emotional support. Mothers, for example, though usually extremely concerned with the child (and often overprotective) derive no pleasure from nursing, and control prevails over tenderness and emotional warmth (Selvini-Palazzoli, 1978).

In an interactional framework in which any possibility of direct expression of emotions and opinions is precluded, the parents' control strategies consist of constantly redefining children's feelings and emotions until they experience them according to the general family pattern. Moreover, this kind of control underlies not only the educational strategies exhibited by parents, but is actually the foundation of a family affectional style that could be phrased: "It is by sharing the same opinions and emotions that we realize we love each other."

One of the most specific invariant aspects of the family inter-action of eating disorder-prone individuals is what Minuchin *et al.* (1978) call "enmeshment":

> Enmeshment refers to an extreme form of proximity and intensity in family interactions. . . . On an individual level, interpersonal differentiation in an enmeshed system is poor. . . . In enmeshed families the individual gets lost in the system. The boundaries that define individual autonomy are so weak that functioning in individually differentiated ways is radically handicapped. . . . Family members intrude on each others' thoughts and feelings. (p. 30)

In such conditions, children develop a deep and pervasive feeling of unreliability concerning their ability to recognize and properly decode their own inner states. Therefore, only within an ongoing emotional relationship with an attachment figure can they infer what is "permissible" to feel and think.

Susan was a 35-year-old travel agent who in early youth had suffered from clear-cut anorexia nervosa that required psychotherapeutic inter-vention.

Her main attachment figure was her father, who was reluctant to permit himself any direct and definite display of emotion. He had impeccable manners, and everybody in the family considered him a model of gentlemanly distinction and elegance. Since early childhood, Susan showed a judicious, mature character, and preferred the company of grown-ups to that of children of her age. Susan's father, who entertained high expectations for her, thought it useless to send her to kindergarten. Thus, at age 5 he put her directly into elementary school, not doubting that she would be able to keep up with older children. Susan could already read and write, and the difficulties that she encountered were, in fact, not connected to learning but rather to socializing with schoolmates and teachers, because she found herself in an entirely new situation. During the first weeks, she seemed a little lost and uncertain, and even her usual composure and calm became less evident for a while.

Susan, however, did not experience the situation as something par-ticularly serious until one day, as she was telling her father about her self doubts about her behavior in class, *she thought she could read on his face* the signs of deep worry. For a second, she panicked at the thought that she was risking the loss of her father's esteem if she overstated her school problems. As she later reported in the course of psychotherapy, this episode was a key experience for Susan. It showed her, on the one hand, that the display of a self-competent attitude was essential for maintaining a preferential relationship with her father; and on the other, that one's problems must, in any case, be kept to oneself.

Brenda's relationship with her mother (see pp. 60, 62, 75) illustrates equally well how a child can scaffold his/her inner states only though an enmeshed relationship with a preferential attachment figure.

Perceived Disappointment within the Preferential Attachment Relationship

In our clinical experience, the developmental pathway of eating disorder-prone individuals seems characterized by a more or less intense experience of disappointment involving the favorite parent. In most cases this occurs sometime between the end of childhood and the adolescent phase (Guidano & Liotti, 1983). Preliminary findings carried out by other investigators have provided confirming evidence regarding these clinical impressions (Hawkins, 1983). While awaiting further controlled prospective–longitudinal studies, I will merely point out the single feature of this experience that, in my opinion, is the most notable.

As discussed in Chapter 4, with the progressive emergence of abstract thought the individual begins to see his/her parents in a totally different way. Although in childhood, and to a greater degree in preschool years, parents were considered the holders of absolute truths and values, with adolescent relativism they are perceived as more or less ordinary people with common uncertainties, contradictions, difficulties, and so on. The change of image is a physiological process and is usually not experienced by adolescents as distressing, because it still supports their emergent sense of individuality while at the same time it begins the process of cognitive–emotional separation from the family.

However, because eating disorder-prone individuals, in order to achieve a stable sense of self, are bound to adhere to the expectations of a parent perceived as an absolute model, a reappraisal of that model obviously can only be experienced as a disappointment—one so intense that it questions one's established sense of self. It could also be stated that within a developmental pathway of this kind, to experience the beginning of the separation process from parents as a reaction to being disappointed in them and to perceive the new emergent feeling of epistemological loneliness as a dreadfully blurred sense of self, is "almost physiological." This probably explains the fact that the experience of disappointment is invariably found in the adolescent reorganization of eating disorder-prone individuals. Indeed, a close examination of these experiences, in spite of their variability, always reveals a common basic element, that is, the relativization of the image of a beloved parent that up to that time was perceived as absolute.

For Susan the disappointment, as fate would have it, resulted from just one of those rare times when she and her father went somewhat beyond their usual formalities and had a moment of greater intimacy. On that occasion, the father, perhaps encouraged by the maturity of the 15-year-old girl whom he now considered a grown woman, revealed to her in the tone of one who is imparting a lesson on the secrets of life, that her mother had become pregnant before marriage. Susan felt extremely upset, although she was able to keep perfectly calm and impassive. Her own words in reporting the episode in therapy can exemplify better than any comment both the nature of the perceived disappointment and the influence the latter had on her subsequent lifespan:

> For days I was unable to look at my mother or my father, but I felt more resentful toward my father. It seemed to me he had deceived me. He had completely betrayed my trust in him. For me the two of them embodied absolute perfection, without the slightest weakness. I guess up to that moment I had thought of them as sexless. I had never imagined before a possible sexual intimacy between them. My father's revelation was upsetting all my theories, and at the same time made me think of him as guilty of the "crime," whereas my mother seemed to be only the victim. . . . A sort of challenge between me and my father has gone on ever since, and is practically endless; it only seems to interrupt at times when I am able to show myself and him that I am autonomous, that I can live even without his approval. . . . It may sound funny, but that was the time when also my sexual problems started.

In Brenda's case, the disappointment is a consequence of the relativization of the image of her mother—as we have seen, her main attachment figure.

Brenda's mother, an attractive, dynamic woman, was very self-confident in her social relations. She always played the role of the person whose interests and aspirations are at a much higher cultural level, but who is being held back in her elan only by the presence of a conservative, old-fashioned husband. She had always told Brenda that a woman should travel, have any number of interests, and, above all, should entirely dedicate herself to her personal realization, almost implying that the relationship with her husband was a burden for her. As a child, Brenda was absolutely sure of all this. She admired her mother and considered her father—who was away most of the time—a stranger or, at most, an undesirable guest.

When Brenda was 13 years old, during one of the rare quarrels between the parents, her usually self-controlled father packed a suitcase and left home, threatening a final separation. Brenda was glad; she thought her mother's secret life dream was finally about to come true. But, as days went by, it became more and more clear that the mother had dropped her usual demeanor, and now appeared crushed and desperate. That was when Brenda realized that the only thing her mother really cared about was to keep her man, and all those interests and beautiful ideas she talked so much about didn't matter at all. She felt completely lost and confused, and at the same time she deemed it her duty now to protect her mother without letting her see that she was aware of her weakness. In the time that followed, Brenda "inexplicably" got fat, until within 2 months she had gained over 30 pounds.

IDENTITY DEVELOPMENT

The interference in the early rhythmical differentiation between self and others seems to be, as we have seen, at the center of the developing child's existing cognitive situation. A psychologically healthy familial attachment style should allow children to achieve a sense of differentiation, while at the same time providing them with an adequate level of emotional identification with the parents. In others words, while clearly perceiving the affective state of a significant attachment figure is a necessary condition for recognizing the same feeling within the self (outward tendency), the acquisition of a definite sense of one's self requires at the same time a turning away from the source of identification (inward tendency). As a consequence, a harmonic interplay between identification and identity processes is based on a dynamic steady balance between the child's outward and inward tendencies. As Minuchin (1974) clearly stated: "Human experience of identity has two elements: a sense of belonging and a sense of being separate. The laboratory in which these ingredients are mixed and dispersed is the family, the matrix of identity" (p. 47).

By continuously preventing children from developing feelings of their own, enmeshed patterns of attachment severely hamper the children's sense of "being separate" and produce during infancy and preschool years a precarious, loose demarcation between their emerging sense of self and the internal representations of parents.

From the earliest stages, the rehearsal of scenes concerning the nonrecognition or disconfirmation of any expression of autonomous feelings and thoughts will bring about the selective differentiation of opponent sets of prototypical emotional schemata as the bases underlying the structuring of a blurred sense of self. As a result, the child's self-boundaries are continuously and loosely wavering between being "externally bound" in order to achieve a definite sense of self (in which the reduced sense of individuality is experienced as a feeling of personal ineffectiveness) and trying to be "internally bound" in defining his/her sense of self (in which the resulting higher sense of individuality is matched by a feeling of emptiness and self-unreliability).

At the end of preschool years, as these prototypical emotional schemata are progressively formalized in a more ordered nuclear scene, children become increasingly able to control their challenging feelings of personal ineffectiveness and emptiness by actively seeking the intermediate states. A steady and dynamic equilibrium is generally achieved by selecting the preferred figure of attachment as the essential "criterion image" for properly decoding one's inner states, while at the same time trying to display self-sufficient, controlled attitudes in order to recover a sense of differentiation from the figure itself. In other words, at a stage when the child should have learned to identify and decode inner states, attention is still completely focused on the parent. As a result, the perception of most impulses and emotions will remain rudimentary and uncertain, with the single remarkable exception of the primitive bodily sensations connected to hunger and motility.

A steady equilibrium of this kind is carried out by specific patterns of decentralized control. On the one hand, the selective exclusion of the sensory inflow capable of activating direct and defined expressions of one's emotions reduces the possibilities of incoming challenging disconfirmations. On the other, by constructing a self-image on the basis of the perceived expectations of the selected parent, the subject can maintain somewhat constant the range of confirmations necessary to stabilize the sense of self. Finally, the variations in bodily sensations like hunger and motility that support the only possibilities of a reliable self-perception are scaffolded into a repertoire of motoric and visceral patterns. These patterns act as diversionary activities aimed at reducing the surfacing into self-consciousness of challenging feelings that convey a sense of personal ineffectiveness and/or emptiness.

These considerations easily explain the tendency toward a pleasing perfection commonly found in the developmental pathway of typical eating disorder-prone children. They are generally good-mannered, apparently maturer than their age, and often successful students. In fact, at least until the disappointment is experienced, the fulfillment of the parent's ideas of perfection is considered the most reliable way of achieving an acceptable level of self-esteem and personal worthiness.

ORGANIZATIONAL ASPECTS

The Adolescent Resolution

The emergence of higher cognitive abilities generally comes with the surfacing of a disequilibrium, for the decentering from the world brought forward by these abilities implies a relativization of the absolute image of the parent on which depended the stable sense of self. The childhood strategy of deriving a definite sense of self from a significant other now is challenged by the distressing discovery of the possibility of being disappointed in such a significant relationship. Therefore the critical feelings of personal ineffectiveness and/or emptiness derived from a blurred and wavering sense of self, in which personal worthiness and self-esteem are vague and indefinite, once again come into the picture.[2]

However, because confirmations coming from significant others are still the essential way of attaining a stable and satisfactory identity, the only possible adolescent resolution is to seek a supportive intimacy and, at the same time, to minimize the effects of disconfirmations and disappointments, whether perceived as the outcome of a deceiving reality or of one's incompetence and unlovableness. The active actor's sense of self coming from the adolescent recentering on oneself can, in fact, vary according to the causal attribution with which the perceived disappointment is scaffolded. Even though the attribution of causality coming from a deep, wavering sense of blurred self always remains within rather ample margins of indefinitess and oscillation, it is still possible to choose, within these margins, an external or internal attribution as a prevailing orientation.

In the case of an external causal attribution, individuals perceive others mainly as deceitful and intrusive. Their commitment to striving against a deceitful reality by strenuously displaying positive, controlled, self-sufficient attitudes, allows them to keep the sense of personal ineffectiveness and emptiness below acceptable limits. During a disequilibrium, this attributional style—involving more active bodily and motoric patterns—can give rise to the typical anorexic disorders.

When an internal attribution is made, the individual's commitment will instead be oriented at restricting the distressing effect of expected disappointments and disconfirmations by attributing them to specific, concrete traits of the self, rather than to the general sense of personal ineffectiveness and emptiness with which he/she feels pervaded. This attributional style, involving more passive bodily and motoric patterns, can in times of disequilibrium be the source of bulimic disorders and obesity.

The establishment of an external rather than internal causal attribution depends on the extent to which the appraisal of the prototypical disappointment is actively "discovered" (i.e., experienced as volitionally imposing one's view upon reality) as opposed to passively "accepted" (i.e., experienced as adapting oneself to an overwhelming distressing event). The developmental variables that may influence the quality of this appraisal can be set out as follows.

1. Intensity of the discrepant event. A challenging situation that overwhelms the child's coping capabilities can, indeed, be only experienced as a passively suffered inescapable concern.

2. The intensity being the same, an important factor is the subject's age when the event is experienced. In the adolescent stage, abstract cognitive abilities allow a more active appraisal as compared to those that occur in childhood. Clinical impressions confirm that in cases of obesity, disappointments usually occurred earlier than in cases of anorexia (Guidano & Liotti, 1983).

3. Intensity and age being the same, a significant factor is the presence or absence of available alternative identification figures

in the child's social network. Up to a certain point, the possibility of replacing a reference model perceived as exclusive with another one, can remarkably contribute to the scaffolding of the ongoing disappointment in the beloved parent as an active cognitive–emotional separation from him/her.

The Attitude toward Oneself and Reality

The eating disorder resolution allows one to achieve a steady and dynamic equilibrium between the absolute need for significant others' confirmations and the impending fear of being disappointed in significant relationships. The recursive oscillation between opponent emotional polarities enables the individual to perceive, on the one hand, a sense of self as reliable and worthy (due to the perceived ability to manipulate others' judgment in his/her favor). On the other, it allows one to recover a sense of individuality and demarcation from others (due to the perceived ability to control their intrusiveness and deceitfulness). This steady and oscillative equilibrium is carried out through the structuring of a specific attitude toward oneself and reality.

The most striking characteristic of the attitude toward oneself is, no doubt, the uncertain attribution of causality with respect to one's feelings and inner states underlying both the perfectionism and the self-deceiving mechanisms typical of eating disorder-prone individuals.

In the process of ordering one's internal experience into an organized whole, the lack of confidence and reliability of one's self-perception exerts a crucial role in molding an overreliance upon external frames of reference. Therefore, if the problem consists of drawing a sense of self out of others' judgments, perfectionism logically becomes the way to provide a positive solution to this problem. As a consequence, one's perceived range of actual and potential self-images is always matched with absolute and conventional standards of perfection, thus starting a cycle of inflationary self-evaluation in which replication of past imagined excellence becomes routinely expected and future endeavours must always set new highs (Mahoney, 1974, pp. 155–156).

This kind of attitude would obviously predispose one to the occurrence of those very disappointments and disconfirmations that would challenge the achieved balance. The perfectionistic attitude, however, is buffered against these challenging perturbations by the parallel structuring of a self-deceiving attitude. This allows one to avoid in advance any possible confrontation that could turn out to be a disappointment or failure, while at the same time selectively excluding the critical feelings of personal ineffectiveness and emptiness from one's felt identity. In other words, it is the uncertain attribution of causality to feelings that makes eating disorder-prone individuals able to prevent themselves from becoming aware of what they actually do know. Brenda's way of defining the relationship with her father is a typical example of this self-deceiving attitude toward oneself: "In point of fact, I never went deeper into the relationship with my father to avoid finding out that I was not his favorite daughter."

The possibility of having an unacceptable body image is the eating disorder-prone individuals' prevailing way of embodying their feelings of personal ineffectiveness and emptiness once the latter have been activated by inevitable or unpredictable challenging confrontations.

Several factors seem to be at the source of this focusing on the body. In the first place, variations in bodily states are still the most reliable impulses for decoding one's ongoing self-perception. Secondly, the family's habit of emphasizing formal and aesthetic aspects of personal identity further contributes to make bodily appearance essential in self-evaluation.[3] Being overweight thus becomes the main way of representing to oneself a possible personal failure. Although the more active, anorexic-prone individuals strive against this image of failure by overcontrolling their biological impulses, obese individuals, on the contrary, tend to give up the struggle, since they feel they are not up to the task.

The eating disorder-prone individual's attitude toward reality shows rather clearly the uncertainties and contradictions with which subjects experience the primacy attributed to the interpersonal realm. On the one side, the attainment of an acceptable sense of self is deemed possible only by establishing an intimate, reciprocal relationship with a significant figure. But on the other, the commitment and self-disclosure necessary to reach this goal inevitably entails the risk of critical judgments or disappointments that would make one's perceived identity even more vague and wavering. Eating disorder-prone individuals' vulnerability to others' negative judgments, in fact, by far exceeds the sensitivity to criticism commonly found in every other P.C.Org. The perception of an unbearable challenge to one's sense of self is well expressed in Susan's description of her feelings when being criticized: "It's a sense of general darkening and dismay, like being under water and sinking deeper and deeper, and your only hope to ever emerge again is to obtain the other person's approval; and that seems more and more unlikely and beyond hope."

In intimate relationships, such a crucial interpersonal dilemma is tentatively resolved through the development of a repertoire of relational strategies aimed at obtaining from the partner the greatest possible guarantee of a supportive intimacy, while avoiding as much as possible any clear commitment and self-exposure in the relationship. However, it is quite obvious that an affectional style characterized by ambiguity, indefiniteness, and constant "testing" of the partner often brings about those very criticisms and disappointments that the individuals fear so much.

SYSTEMIC COHERENCE

In a systemic perspective, the primacy of nuclear scenes concerning a hindered sense of one's individuality immediately stands out when we consider the central role attributed to the interpersonal domain both in the development and in the organization of an eating disorder P.C.Org. Moreover, as the emergence of logical/deductive thinking brings forth disappointments, the role attributed to interpersonal domain initially undergoes a relativization. Subsequently, the search for supportive relationships turns into a more complex attitude, aimed at obtaining a confirmation of one's felt identity while, at the same time, preserving the gradually emerging sense of one's individuality.

As previously discussed, the steady and dynamic equilibrium attained in adolescence and youth has its own internal contradictions and discrepancies; the most noteworthy in the eating disorders attitude toward oneself and reality is the ability to produce events apt to be easily scaffolded in terms of disconfirmations and disappointments.

However, it is through the very assimilation and integration of the distressing feelings activated by these disequilibria that individuals have a chance to reach more structured and reliable patterns of self-perception during their temporal becoming. In other words, this is a knowing strategy whose directionality is expressed through a progressive relativization of others and matched by a growing sense of individuality and personal autonomy. This directionality, in turn, can be regarded as an ongoing, emerging product resulting from the moment-to-moment unfolding of the pattern of organizational closure underlying the systemic coherence of an eating disorder P.C.Org.—that is, the fact that one's inner life becomes progressively ordered into personal experience only if matched with the recursive oscillation between the need for others' approval and the fear of being intruded upon or disappointed by others.

Of course, the experience-assimilating procedures of the "anorexic" are different from the "obese" eating disorder pattern. In the former case, the active struggle to keep control over one's perceived personal ineffectiveness often leads to the structuring of more complex and abstract self-sufficient attitudes. Thus, the way Susan made her choice of a professional career during her last high school year fairly exemplifies how the scaffolding of a new attitude that makes alternative experiential domains available can be the result of an active reaction to a perceived disappointment.

After she had felt disappointed by her father and until she was about 19 years old, Susan had several short love affairs with young men that she herself described as dull and mediocre. During that time, she had carefully avoided becoming too involved with a classmate she really liked, who had been dating her insistently for some time. During the last school year, this young man had a motorcycle accident and had to spend a few weeks in the hospital. Susan began to visit him every afternoon, out of a sense of friendship and solidarity. Actually, she felt protected by this circumstance. It allowed her to provide a definition (however vague and ambiguous) to her true feelings for him without forcing her into a clear self-exposure and affective commitment. At the same time, it allowed her to increasingly test how her visits were becoming essential to him.

It was a time of elation for Susan, but it came to an end as soon as he was well again and left the hospital. Although he was still affectionate and kind to her, he returned to other friendships and usual activities, and Susan felt deeply disappointed in no longer being at the center of his attention. In a short while, and in spite of the young man's continued affectionate approaches, Susan again developed the cool, detached attitude that she had had before the accident. This experience, however, made Susan realize how her self-esteem and competence were deeply connected to a sense of feeling needed by someone—so much so that, when school finished, she decided to enroll in medical school.

In the "obese" pattern, the more passive attitude toward distressing feelings activated by a disappointment often leads to the structuring of bodily and emotional patterns that may provide more defined and controllable forms to one's perceived personal ineffectiveness. The way Brenda let the relationship with her boyfriend end is a good example of how even a passive, internal causal attribution can lead to the relativization of a significant other.

At age 18, Brenda had a sense of growing uncertainty about her relationship with her first boyfriend. Because her mother objected to it, Brenda was afraid of losing her approval and thus felt more and more uneasy about his requests for a greater involvement on her part, while at the same time she was afraid of bringing her femininity into question if she refused. Indeed, the image she had of her boyfriend—one of the brightest and most brilliant in her class—was one of almost absolute perfection. In this situation of uncertainty, her sense of personal ineffectiveness grew to the point of producing panic attacks, in one case so intense as to cause a loss of consciousness (see p. 75).

One day, while he was explaining to her his ideal of womanly beauty, the boy, teasing her affectionately, told Brenda that if she got just a little plumper he would be forced to leave her. Brenda didn't seem to take the remark too seriously, but in a short time and without knowing why, she gained almost 10 pounds. She obviously felt deeply disappointed by the young man's reaction of progressive detachment and realized only then how wrong she had been in thinking highly of a man who gave so much importance to physical appearance.

THE DYNAMICS OF COGNITIVE DYSFUNCTION

Within the eating disorder-prone individual's search for a self-directed identity, a disequilibrium is generally the result of the activation of distressing feelings of personal ineffectiveness and/or emptiness. Because of their difficulty in assimilating and integrating such feelings, individuals are led to explain and control them through modifications of their body image produced by alterations of the eating behavior.

Life events likely to activate such challenging pressures can be subsumed into two main groups.

1. *Changes in an interpersonal relationship that the subject perceives as extremely meaningful.* This often occurs when an unpleasant discovery or revelation is made about an attachment figure that forces a sudden reassessment of both the person and the relationship. As we have seen in the case of both Susan and Brenda, this is one of the mechanisms that most frequently initiates the first adolescent disappointment. In other instances, demands for a clearer and more defined commitment and for self-exposure within the relationship are experienced as too challenging. Finally, another rather common situation concerns the onset of a true crisis in a long-lasting intimate relationship, in which the subject feels that it is impossible either to leave the partner or to accept being deserted by him/her.

2. *Developmental changes or new environmental demands that produce a confrontation with a new situation that the subject perceives as an unbearable challenge to his/her established sense of self-competence.* The adolescent maturation, coupled with consequent separation from the family and new psychosocial adjustments, is most certainly a crucial stage in the eating disorders developmental pathway. Indeed, anorexia nervosa has been considered since the beginning a typical adolescent syndrome. Disappointments or disconfirmations that can elicit a disequilibrium in this critical period can often go unnoticed by an outside observer because they frequently involve very common situations like teasing comments from peers that are in no way different from what other adolescents hear about having curves or being chunky (Bruch, 1978).

Finally, other circumstances that can easily be perceived as challenging "testing benches" for one's established sense of self-competence concern either highly valued measures of success in one's social environment—such as final high-school examinations, graduations, and so on—or changes in family or work responsibilities requiring an increased and more defined commitment.

A disequilibrated eating disorder P.C.Org. is characterized by an interplay among simultaneous and competing processes. On the one hand, the emergence of critical feelings that challenge one's ongoing felt identity increases a blurred sense of self. On the other, there is the attempt to exclude such feelings from one's felt identity (or at least to control them) by attributing them to circumscribed parts of the self. The interplay between these processes can be outlined as follows.

1. At the conscious level, the pervasive feeling of personal ineffectiveness takes form in the unbearable representation of having an unacceptable body image, usually corresponding to the image of a figure made shapeless by fat.

In the anorexic pattern, this image is fought against through a strained control of one's biological impulses—so much so that the struggle often becomes saliently paradoxical. The subjects keep seeing themselves fat, although they are near starvation due to reduced and whimsical eating, spontaneous or self-provoked vomiting, misuse of laxatives, and diuretics, and so forth. The level of motor activity is generally exalted and in keen contrast to a worn-out physical appearance. The anorexic attempt to maintain a consistent positive self-image is carried out by opposing the challenging sense of ineffectiveness with a sense of a personal power derived from the continuous confirming experience of being able to dominate even the deepest and most embedded impulses. As Selvini-Palazzoli (1978) noted, for the anorexic client, every victory over the flesh is, at the same time, a confirmation of a greater control over one's biological impulses and a "magic key" to a greater power.

In the obese pattern, conversely, individuals grow exceedingly fat (either by constant overeating, or by intermittent eating binges or bulimic attacks), and think themselves totally unable to control their impulses. The level of motoric activity is usually extremely low. Because of the prevailing internal causal attribution, the effort to keep the accustomed self-image unaltered as much as possible consists, in this case, of accepting one's perceived negativity, but restricting it solely to external appearance. The diversionary role played by this passivity and lack of control is, indeed, clearly highlighted by what could be rightly considered a catchword of obese people: "What other people reject is not really me; they reject my fat body."

2. At the tacit level, the motor setting and autonomic activation that accompany the arousal of the critical feelings of personal ineffectiveness and emptiness, in the absence of an adequate cognitive mediation, tend to be directly realized without any delay or control in the corresponding alterations of the eating and motoric patterns.

Over time, the trend of an eating disorder cognitive dysfunction shows a certain degree of diversity between anorexic and obese patterns. As a rule, anorexia represents an acute disequilibrium of the adolescent/youth phase, and consequently exhibits a certain tendency toward readjustment. This is most likely to occur when—through psychotherapy or intervening changes—interpersonal situations responsible for the critical experiences of disappointment or disconfirmation are modified or removed. Optimum situations are obviously those in which the readjustment coincides with an adequate integration of the disequilibrium leading to a progressive shift in self-awareness.

In contrast, obesity—especially when its onset occurs during adulthood—exhibits a certain tendency to structure itself in a rather stable self-deceiving attitude aimed at coping with both one's perceived negativity and others' deceitfulness and intrusiveness. In other words, the more it becomes clear that one's failure could consist of not being loved and approved, the more the subject can feel that an unacceptable physical appearance is what protects him/her from further intolerable disappointments or rejections.

NOTES

1. Altan is an Italian cartoonist whose strips in recent years have acquired great popularity because of their psychological penetration and attention to current social realities.

2. Because the most outstanding problem in an eating disorder adolescent resolution is to provide an integrated and defined form to a blurred and wavering sense of self, it can be reasonably suggested that the difficulties in reaching such an integrated self can manifest themselves by disturbances that could classically be labeled as psychotic. In fact, many traditional psychiatrists, in the face of an "identity crisis" like the one Brenda experienced at the age of 18 (see p. 75), would strongly suspect the existence of a possible underlying psychotic process.

3. The role of social and cultural factors in attributing personal worth to body appearance is certainly remarkable. In regard to this matter it may be interesting to relate clinical observations collected in one of the most isolated and traditionally backward regions of Italy—Sardinia. Up until a few years ago, when conditions in the island were still almost feudal, anorexia was virtually nonexistent. In the system of values of an archaic peasant society, the body was considered only a natural medium between the person and the world and an instrument of survival with which most people established a relationship of necessity, free of any aesthetic dimension. Only recently, with the advent of radical economic, cultural, and social changes, have anorexia cases gradually become more frequent in Sardinia.

CHAPTER TEN

THE OBSESSIVE COGNITIVE ORGANIZATION

Not doubt, but certainty leads to madness. —Musil

The organizational unity of obsessive-prone individuals' emotional domain rests on a perceived ambivalent and dichotomous sense of self unfolding through antithetical boundaries of meaning oscillating in an "all-or-none" manner. Thus any disequilibrium in one's need for absolute certainty is immediately experienced as a total lack of control. The experience of uncontrollability is matched by the surfacing of behaviors, images, and thoughts that persist unnecessarily and in spite of one's intentions, and that are therefore perceived as distressing self–alien products (Adams, 1973; Beech, 1974; Guidano & Liotti, 1983; Salzman, 1973). We shall begin, as usual, by directing our attention to the developmental processes at the base of the systemic coherence exhibited by the obsessive pattern of organizational closure.

INVARIANT ASPECTS OF DYSFUNCTIONAL PATTERNS OF ATTACHMENT

The central feature of the developmental pathway of an obsessive P.C.Org. concerns the elaboration of an ambivalent sense of self resulting from dysfunctional patterns of familial attachment.

Regardless of the various forms that it may take, the abnormal course of attachment relationships with parents can be referred to by a constellation of invariant aspects that, though generally present, combine with each other in different ways from case to case. The most common seem to be as follows.

1. *Ambivalent patterns of attachment.* The parenting behavior of at least one of the caregivers (the other is usually a minor, relatively insignificant figure) is characterized by mixed and opposite feelings

toward the child; a rejecting, hostile attitude is concealed and camouflaged by an outward facade of devotion and concern. Furthermore, the level of feeling display and emotional warmth of the attachment relationship is mostly very low (Adams, 1973; Barnett, 1966; Laughlin, 1967).

A simple, schematic situation is one in which a parent, though attentive and totally dedicated to the child's moral and social education, never expresses his/her love with tenderness or other affective displays. The *simultaneousness* of these contradictory aspects in parenting behavior seems to be an important prerequisite for the obsessive developmental pathway. As an example of such simultaneousness, imagine a parent talking to his/her child about parental love being one of the most important values in the world while keeping his/her face rigid and expressionless and showing no emotion.

In most cases, however, more frankly hostile attitudes are continuously intermingled with expressions of care and protection, giving the child a sense of uncontrollability and unpredictability about rewards and punishments in his/her fundamental attachment relationships.

Alison was a 29-year-old secretary who, in late adolescence, had suffered from obsessive disorders that had required psychotherapy.

Alison's mother, her primary attachment figure, was a cold, aloof woman who considered physical contacts as mere useless, even unhealthy sentimentalities. She had strict moral standards, and personally took care of her daughter's upbringing (to which she dedicated most of her time). Beginning around the time of Alison's preschool years, this constant attention was shown, however, only through a continuous repetition of rigid rules of conduct that admitted no exception, and through requests for detailed explanations of the reasons for even the slightest little disobedience (which Alison, at that age, was absolutely unable to give). Upset by what she regarded as reticence, the mother would then close herself in worried silences that could last for several days. For example, Alison remembered clearly how every day she waited for the time to come home from school with a mixture of wishful anticipation and anguish. On the one hand, after a whole day away from home, she was anxious to be with her mother again, and she felt her mother shared her desire, because she usually left whatever she was doing to meet her. But, on the other hand, as soon as they were together, the mother would start reproaching her endlessly about her dust-covered shoes, her dirty hands, her wrinkled dress and so on.

Later on, as an adult, Alison commented about these episodes in a way that clearly expressed her feeling that her mother's behavior was totally unpredictable: "What I never could understand is whether my mother really loved me or not. I knew that if she took so much care of me it had to mean she loved me, but she seemed to be doing it only to reproach me. Anyhow, it was a constant strain for me, it was like feeling always "under fire.""

Another instance of attachment showing simultaneously two antithetic aspects—in this case love at the tacit level and rejection at the explicit one—has been reported in the case of Derek (see p. 73).

Ambivalent attachments of the kind described above closely resemble a communicative situation in which it is objectively impossible not to choose, but in which any choice is *logically* wrong, that is, a "double-bind" situation (Bateson, Jackson, Haley, & Weakland, 1956). While the double-bind hypothesis was at first regarded to be of major importance in the pathogenesis of schizophrenia, in recent years it has been increasingly considered to be a universal pathogenic mechanism in a wide variety of abnormal behaviors (Sluzki & Veron, 1976). The specificity of an obsessive developmental pathway, therefore, should not be explained solely by the presence of ambivalent attachments but rather by their being in combination with the following other anomalies of the obsessive family environment.

2. *Predominance of digital and analytical over analogical and immediate forms of communication.* The households of obsessive families are usually highly verbal, with parents who are motorically underactive but verbally hyperactive (Adams, 1973). In such conditions, all spontaneousness and naturalness is stifled by the parents' constant devaluation of any physical activity and their unwillingness to take part in and encourage the children's participation in games, except, of course, in the case of educational or intellectual games.

Within this highly verbal environment, which lacks tenderness and emotional warmth, parents' constant pressing for absolute love and affection from the child results in the child's expressions of affection and emotion becoming more and more paradoxical and disturbed (Salzman, 1973). In fact, the best display of affection comes to coincide with what would appear to be its opposite, that is, serious, pensive, and detached behavior.

One of Derek's sharpest memories concerned an afternoon he had gone shopping with his mother. He was 5 years old, and had begun elementary school a few months earlier. It was Christmas time and Derek walked composedly beside his mother, showing little or no curiosity about the cheerful atmosphere and the inviting decorations in the store windows. It was one of those none too frequent days when he had not yet been reproached by his mother, and he did not want to in any way perturb this situation, being fully aware that his mother would not approve of his childish curiosities and enthusiasms. All of a sudden, taking Derek completely by surprise, his mother stopped and in her usual removed manner told him that since he had behaved and done well in school, he deserved a present and could look around and choose whatever he liked. Derek at once felt a surge of affection for his mother, but he remained perfectly controlled and impassive, and in a serious, pensive manner answered that the present he would appreciate most was a book.

If we stop to imagine the usual feelings and behavior of a child who is unexpectedly offered whatever he likes among a whole feast of Christmas presents, we can get an idea of the lack of spontaneousness and naturalness that an obsessive-prone child exhibits in his/her attachment relationships.

3. Finally, family style and parental attitudes assume, in their whole, all the characteristics of a *truly unreasonably demanding environment for the child* (Salzman, 1973). After an early phase of overindulgence corresponding to physical caregiving, parents in obsessive families become extremely demanding for maturity and responsibility, seeing in the child simply a miniature adult. Strong emphasis upon moral values and ethical principles—rather than on the expression of genuine religious or spiritual ideals—is usually an instrument used by parents to obtain virtually total control over the child's conduct and emotions.

Thus, typically all feelings that seem incompatible with such values (anger, sexuality, and so on) are absolutely "forbidden." It is never said that these feelings should be controlled, but rather, that they are *not* to be felt at all. Since emotions, by their nature, are unavoidable and unescapable, this inevitably becomes an additional, paradoxical experience of uncontrollability for the child.

Finally, by invoking arguments such as sense of responsibility and the need for sacrifice in order to face responsibilities, it becomes possible to control children's entire conduct, rewarding them only for the efforts they make and not for the results they obtain. "Nothing is freely provided; all must be earned by effort; and love itself is doled out as merited" (Adams, 1973, p. 64).

IDENTITY DEVELOPMENT

Being at the center of the early, existing cognitive situation, the experience of a "double*f*aced" attachment in which opposite and antithetical feelings are incompatibly mixed, deeply influences— via the "looking-glass effect"—the child's unfolding processes of self-recognition.

On the one hand, the image of an all-giving, apparently overindulgent parent will be matched by the elaboration of emotional schemata that convey the sense of reliability of the outside world and of one's own acceptability. But on the other, the simultaneous experiencing of the same parent as demanding, controlling, and rejecting will produce opposite emotional schemata in which the sense of one's unacceptability will be tinged with feelings of anger and hostility. Paraphrasing the unsolvable dilemma tacitly perceived by the child, it could be said that the experiences "He/she loves me; I am lovable" and "He/she loves me not; I am unlovable" both have evidence in their favor and explain equally well the same ongoing attachment relationship.

Therefore, ever since the earliest stages of development, the emergence of split patterns of self-recognition will be matched by the structuring of an oscillative recursive loop in which opposite and antithetical feelings come to be organized into a regulation process based exclusively on their mutual and reciprocal exclusion, thus strongly reducing the possibilities of reaching a single, integrated self-perception. In other terms, while, for example, a depressive-prone child (and the same goes for all other P.C.Orgs.) has a sense of self based on both opponent polarities of sadness and anger, the obsessive child, in order to have a reliable sense of self, is forced to rely each time only on *one* of the antithetic polarities, that is, either he/she is lovable and acceptable, or he/she is neither.

These abrupt oscillations between opposite and incompatible emotional experiences can be perceived without serious consequences during the early self-centered infancy, but with the advent of higher decentering abilities due to the development of concrete cognitive capacities, they will start being scaffolded into discrepant and distressing experiences of self-perception. An accurate reconstruction of the preschool period of obsessive-prone individuals frequently reveals bizarre and frightening "insights" about oneself that are not generally found in previously described P.C.Orgs.

Derek remembered clearly the time he had begun to mistrust and fear his own imagination. He was about 5 or 6 years old, and from a window of his home he was looking at a large oak tree in the garden. He watched it and immediately closed his eyes to see if he was able to imagine it exactly as he had seen it a second before. He was probably at his first steps on the long pathway that leads to the discovery that imagination is a property of thought and not a constitutive element of "objective" reality. While he marveled at finding that no difference actually existed between the real tree and the imagined one, he was suddenly struck by the pervading and painful sense that he himself could be nothing but an image in somebody's mind. He interrupted the game at once and with his usual composure joined his mother in the kitchen. However, even as he grew up, he always considered this episode as one of the strongest and most awkward in his childhood.

At any rate, it is also due to the emergence of cognitive abilities that the ensembles of antithetical emotional schemata can be formalized in a more ordered nuclear scene with which the child becomes more and more able to control his/her opposite patterns of self-perception by actively selecting one of them. A steady and dynamic equilibrium will thus become tentatively achievable only as far as the perceiving of oneself as capable of fulfilling others' requirements becomes the essential "criterion image" for decoding one's felt identity as acceptable and worthwhile (Adams, 1973; Salzman, 1973).

However, in order to maintain the reliability of one's selected self-image, it becomes necessary to exclude and control the constant surfacing of mixed feelings resulting from the tacit experiencing of one's ambivalent self-boundaries. Favored by the deficient development of the analogical understanding (due to having grown in an almost exclusively verbal family environment) obsessive-prone children, therefore, become selectively inattentive to the modulation provided by their inner states—privileging thought and linguistic capabilities to the point of making them their only instrument for understanding reality. In fact, while images and emotions are analogical processes that supply an even number of conflicting data in an immediate and tacit way, verbal processes appear to be more easily controllable, as their digital–sequential format allows one to distribute information into two distinctly differentiable opposites and to make certain, precise choices.

Moreover, this need for certainty, demonstrated by the tendency to adhere to an established order and expressing the child's struggle to maintain a reliable self-identity, is constantly confirmed and oriented further by the parents' attitude. A strict, very orderly parent with an inflexible attitude on duties, values, and responsibilities may support the idea that there are absolute certainties in the world, and that it is absolutely necessary to seek them out and behave according to them.

Patterns of decentralized control apt to maintain the attained dynamic equilibrium will be based, therefore, on this "primacy of the verbal." Thus, through the selective exclusion of free fantasy, imagery, emotions, and impulses it is possible to reduce substantially the surfacing in consciousness of mixed, ambivalent feelings. Should the challenging feelings emerge nonetheless, a whole repertoire of diversionary activities will effectively divert one's conscious attention from further processing them. These activities mainly take on the form of thoughts (ruminations, doubting, etc.) and stereotyped behaviors (rituals), since in the concrete stage of childhood motoric patterns are the prevailing and usual way of controlling the unfolding of cognitive abilities.

Within a developmental pathway completely oriented toward acquiring the certainty of one's felt identity through the exclusion of one's emotional life, the obsessive-prone individual toward the end of childhood will progressively assume the features of a boy or girl whose lack of naturalness and spontaneousness is counterbalanced by a remarkable verbal fluency and linguistic competence, and whose sense of personal worth is intertwined with feelings of omnipotence of thought.

ORGANIZATIONAL ASPECTS

The Adolescent Resolution

The childhood strategies for maintaining a reliable felt identity are challenged by the emergence of higher cognitive abilities, as the differentiation of a reflective dimension of consciousness now allows a more continuous surfacing of mixed, ambivalent feelings. The active actor's sense of self resulting from the adolescent's recentering on him/herself makes the individual perceive as a weakness any recognition of ambivalent feelings and attitudes. Therefore, the striving to attain a reliable perception of oneness will be matched by a commitment to certainty in any domain of experience.

Turning a "double-faced" experiencing of self into its opposite, namely, into a unitary and stable, and preferably positive self-image, necessarily implies that one's pervasive feeling of ambivalence is constantly matched by the opposite procedure—that is, to feel and think exclusively by way of opposite categories and to pass from one to the other in an "all-or-none" way so that unless the achievement of an illusive certainty gives him/her a sense of total control, the individual tends to experience a total lack of control (Salzman, 1973). As can be noticed, the struggle for a defined, unitary identity underlies both the adolescent resolution, and the subsequent adult organization of an obsessive-prone individual. In fact, through the adoption of an all-or-none procedure, he/she can obtain, in any case, an absolute and consequently certain perception of self and reality, with the only difference being that in the one case it will be a positive and in the other a negative one.

The attribution of causality will vary in an all-or-none way depending on the individual's experience. In the positive dimension, an external causal attribution will prevail, and the need for certainty will be expressed by constant activity aimed at foreseeing and anticipating any possible unexpected event brought about by a deceiving, untrustworthy reality. In the negative dimension, conversely, the pervasive sense of an inherent and uncontrollable negativity of the self is the prevailing way in which an internal causal attribution will try to control and explain the challenging feelings emerging as a result of discrepant ongoing experience.

The Attitude toward Oneself and Reality

The adolescent commitment to certainty therefore permits one to reach a unitary and definite self-identity through a steady and dynamic equilibrium oscillating solely between the extreme, antithetic dimensions of controllability and uncontrollability, both experienced as absolute.

This steady oscillation between dichotomous dimensions of meaning is highlighted, at the level of the attitude toward oneself, by the antithetic opposition between thinking and feeling. Because the perception of a unitary identity is equated with the perceived certainty of having total control of oneself, the overconfidence in thought and intellectuality represents the preferential device for attaining a rigid control over one's emotions. By regarding only the rational and logic aspects of one's ongoing self-perception as worthy of attention and further processing, it actually becomes possible to exclude mixed, ambivalent feelings that would lead to a challenging sense of weakness. This would also serve to prevent other feelings such as hostility, anger, and sexuality that would produce feelings of shame, incompetence, and unworthiness. The childish and juvenile sense of omnipotence of thought, transformed by the adolescent overemphasis on abstract thinking, gradually structures itself in a tendency to assume omniscience. Thus, the individual, anticipating and being prepared for anything, feels sure that he/she will have, in all cases, the right reactions (Salzman, 1973).

The constant search to be certain of having the right reaction is further supported by a perfectionistic attitude by which the subject adheres to a rigid set of moral standards and rules, even in the most everyday situations. This sort of perfectionism is, however, seldom actualized in one's actual life program, for the sense of being a positive and firm person depends almost exclusively on the *formal adhering* to moral rules perceived as absolute certainties. As a consequence, perfectionism is expressed by seeking justice, equity, truth and so on, for their own sake with little correlation to the irreducibly unique aspects of the ongoing concrete situation.

It goes without saying that an equilibrium based on a search for certainty carried out solely through cognitive modes has its own internal contradictions and discrepancies.

One of the most typical is the tendency to fractionate ongoing experience, dwelling excessively on its constituent details and failing to envisage the whole. The relative incapability to reach an overall vision of an ongoing situation is undoubtly ascribed to the selective nonuse of global, apprehensional frames supplied by the emotion–imagery mechanism. The predominance given to detail—the so called obsessive "underinclusion" (Reed, 1969)—is expressed in a sort of inability to reach a decision whenever the situation presents some complexity. The perceived difficulty in deciding, in turn, is one of the conditions in which it is most likely that a challenging sense of weakness may be felt, due to the surfacing of mixed and ambivalent feelings.

Furthermore, because the control of emotions is directed at a rigid exclusion of any emotional–imaginative modulation, the individual has a tendency to experience even the slightest feelings that escape his/her control as extremely intense, with the consequent tendency to unduly overreact. The possibility of perceiving oneself as at the mercy of one's own emotions, in turn, increases the probability of the surfacing of challenging feelings such as shame and unworthiness.

As a response to these possible discrepancies and due to the presence of nonarticulate, opposite negative and positive self-images, the subject is able to keep under control the challenging feelings by displacing in an all-or-none way his/her causal attribution toward an internally perceived negativity. This "attributional shift" temporally dislocates these opposite self-images, so that the negative "actual" self is matched by the positivity of a "potential" self perceived as possible in a near future (Makhlouf-Norris, Gwynne-Jones, & Norris, 1970; Makhlouf-Norris, & Norris, 1972). In other words, the subject can maintain a negative but certain identity in actuality, while at the same time preventing his/her self-esteem from decreasing below individual tolerance limits.

Because the primary concern for the obsessive-prone individual is essentially based on safeguarding a unitary sense of self through the adhesion to formal moral rules, the attitude toward reality is characterized, as a general rule, by the relatively low emphasis on others and their way of understanding experience. Moreover, considering that all the unitarity depends on the sense of total control of oneself and that, because of the developmental history, problems arise in giving and receiving tenderness and emotional warmth, the possibilities of a genuine commitment and emotional involvement are, understandably, reduced. Also in relationships with significant others, the obsessional all-or-none attitude is revealed by a formal and rigid dichotomization of any interpersonal experience into opposite aspects, so as to be certain of pursuing the positive aspects and carefully avoiding the negative ones. Doubting, procrastination, and overconcern for details accompany every significant situation of one's affectional life—marriage, pregnancy, childbirth, divorce, etc.—in order to avoid any possible mistake or danger and to find the "certain," "right" attitude to face them.

In other terms, systematic doubting becomes the preferred strategy for reaching a unitary and reliable experiencing of reality. The paradox is, however, quite evident. The highly valued certainty for which the individual so relentlessley strives leads to doubt about everything, and thus inflicts severe blows to his/her certainties. The resulting doubtful, pedantic attitude is, usually, in keen contrast to the individual's linguistic competence and verbal fluency. The remarkable rhetoric abilities and the emphasis placed upon accuracy and completeness are, in fact, the preferential way in which obsession-prone individuals try to control their perception of doubts and uncertainties and, at the same time, cope with the criticism of others that they resent so much (Turner, Steketee, & Foa, 1979).

SYSTEMIC COHERENCE

In a systemic perspective, the primary role exerted by nuclear scenes conveying an ambivalent, double-faced sense of self is highlighted by the fact that the striving to attain a unitary and stable identity is the main thread around which revolve both the development and the organization of an obsessive P.C.Org. In a situation in which a steady, double-bind emotional attachment is the basis for the undecodability of one's feelings, *thought*—in its concrete, and subsequently in its abstract, forms—represents the only possibility of constructing a reliable and defined self. Therefore, during childhood, the individual is able to concretely circumscribe a more defined sense of self through a rigid control of emotions. Later, with adolescence and youth, the ordering of experience into a single, certain, and absolute image of reality provides certainty and consistency to the gradually circumscribed sense of self.

But, as we have seen, the core of the attained equilibrium is composed of a series of discrepancies that can upset the balance at any time. On the one hand, the indispensable search for certainty is constantly undermined by that very process of systematic doubting used to achieve it. On the other hand, the excessive control over inner states inevitably produces the surfacing of feelings and intrusive images experienced as uncontrollable, that challenge the attained unitary self-image.

The intermittent emergence of uncontrollable feelings that challenge one's need for certainty and the subsequent attempts to assimilate them and integrate them are the foundation of the generativity and directionality exhibited by an obsessive cognitive strategy. In fact, such directionality should be expressed in the course of one's lifespan by a progressive relativization of the image of an absolute reality—matched by the emergence of an irreducible sense of one's personal uniqueness and based on a more adequate perception and decoding of one's inner states. In simpler words, it could be said that an obsessive-prone individual should come to discover that the sense of a sure personal identity cannot rely on the impersonal universality of thought, but rather on the perceived uniqueness of his/her personal emotional domain.

The fact that within such directionality one's emotional life is progressively scaffolded into one's felt identity only through a sequence of personal crises and readjustments stemming from the all-or-none, positive–negative, recursive oscillation, represents the pattern of organizational closure underlying the systemic coherence of an obsessive P.C.Org. As an example, let us consider the way in which Alison at age 16 came to recognize that sexual impulses and desires were part of herself.

After puberty, sexuality had become for Alison another critical domain to be controlled with diffidence and aloofness. About that time she attended the wedding of a cousin who had married when she was already pregnant. The fact in itself impressed Alison and aroused in her doubts and perplexities, but what struck her most was a comment her mother had made. With a serious look, she told Alison that it wasn't right to behave like her cousin, who had allowed herself to become pregnant without even being sure she loved her prospective husband. To Alison this meant that a lack of control over one's sexual impulses—which to her meant being no less than a prostitute—was something that could happen to anyone—even her. By the look in her mother's eyes, she seemed to be hinting that the experience was *especially possible* for Alison, that is, that she could, even unwillingly, be a prostitute. At once Alison changed her behavior; she became stiff and austere and denied herself anything (make up, clinging clothes, and so on) that might stress the bodily changes she had gone through. Probably for these reasons, the boys in her class started teasing her, cracking jokes that she could not understand and that increased her doubts and uncertainties. The situation suddenly worsened when one of these boys, alone with her in the school garden, repeatedly made sexual advances. What Alison found most disquieting was not the episode in itself (since her mother had already warned her not to trust boys) but the fact that the "fight" in which she was unwillingly involved had aroused in her new and upsetting sensations.

Immediately she was flooded with intrusive images of an obscene nature that eluded her controlling capacity and were matched by the obsessive, hammering fear that she could be a prostitute. The only possible solution to her doubting was to check her new disturbing sensations over and over, to be certain about what she felt. Masturbation soon began to assume the features of a check and recheck activity, and after a first period of causing distress and guilt, it seemed to have an appeasing effect. It made her feel that the regulation of sexual impulses followed more or less the same rules as all other physiological impulses.

An intense all-or-none oscillation from the image of a positive, controlled person to the image of a prostitute, and the consequent final readjustment was, therefore, what enabled Alison to structure into an emotionally charged personal domain what for most people is simply an ordinary physiological experience, namely, learning that masturbation is the simplest and most immediate way to know and control one's sexual impulses.

This is similar to Derek's experience (see p. 73); the control he progressively acquired at the age of 20 during his distressing checkings and recheckings about the certainty that his involvement with the partner would be everlasting corresponded to a deepening and further personalizing of an already acquired emotional domain. His doubts, concerning only abstract and absolute categories of love, faded away as he became conscious that the variety of emotions experienced in his relationship with a young woman (attraction, jealousy, resentment, etc.) all pertained to different shades of the same feeling of attachment.

The possibilities of assimilating disequilibria will, of course, vary according to the specific developmental pathway and the level of complexity in the concreteness–abstractness dimension attained by the individual. In cases in which the emergence of a personal crisis gives way to a clear-cut clinical syndrome preventing an adequate final readjustment, the lifespan tendency toward the achievement of a full sense of personal uniqueness will inevitably encounter interferences and distortions.

THE DYNAMICS OF COGNITIVE DYSFUNCTION

The steady and dynamic equilibrium of an obsessive P.C.Org. can be unbalanced to the point of producing a clear-cut clinical syndrome by a series of life events that nullify the individual's rigid search for certainty, thus allowing the feared mixed, ambivalent feelings to emerge. In other words, the ease with which apparently irrelevant episodes initiate the process of disequilibrium can account for the inconsistencies among the numerous studies concerned with precipitating life events and obsessive cognitive dysfunction (cf. Black, 1974). Life events most frequently found, however, invariably correspond to emotionally charged situations in which it is difficult to discriminate—according to the individual's standards—between "positive" and "negative" opposite aspects. Thus, it becomes increasingly difficult to reach an adequate comprehension of the situation and consequently to make decisions; the surfacing of challenging feelings is intensified, as is the painful sense of uncontrollability connected to them.

These situations can roughly be summarized as: (1) interpersonal problems in a significant relationship (sexual difficulties, marital crises, etc.); (2) pregnancy and childbirth; (3) separation, loss, or illness of a near relative or someone close; (4) disappointments or failures in the professional life, or overwork.

A disequilibrated obsessive P.C.Org. is characterized by an interplay between simultaneous and competing processes. On the one side, the emergence of intrusive images intermingled with mixed, ambivalent feelings challenge one's striving to maintain the selected unitary, positive felt identity. On the other, individuals, with their typical all-or-none procedure, will try through repetitious, devastating thoughts and behavior patterns, to achieve at least the certainty of being able to control and circumscribe their perceived negativity.

The interplay between these processes can be sketched out as follows.

1. At the conscious level, the attempt to control the challenging feelings is carried out according to the principle of the "primacy of the verbal" characteristic of the obsessive cognitive organization.

Recurring, dominating thoughts (ruminations, doubting, checks and rechecks, and so on), due to the developmental connection between thoughts and actions, are matched by specific sequences of behavior and are structured in true *rituals* that vary from case to case and are peculiar to each individual. Rituals are repetitive activities, sometimes stereotyped, frequently interwoven with superstitious or magic representations of controlling powers. Though employed for the purpose of controlling imagined dangers, rituals actually become serious threats to the individual's very happiness and efficiency. Finally, these activities, however useless and distressing, as the subjects themselves often admit, are compulsively enacted with such scrupulousness and search for perfection that they become the prevailing concern in life. Rituals, therefore, effectively highlight the typical obsessional striving to attain total control of oneself and the environment, and, in the final analysis, the need to reach a certainty of one's perceived negativity and its possible consequences.

Striving for total control and looking for an ultimate certainty are the thematic contents at the core of the diversionary activities with which subjects prevent themselves from further processing and acquiring full awareness of their emotions. "Rather than face an awareness of the impossibility of being omniscient and acknowledging his human limitations, the obsessional concludes that if only he knew more and tried harder he could achieve these goals. The solution is to become more perfect, and thus even more obsessional" (Salzman, 1973, p. 23). In this way, the obsessive concern becomes absolute and takes on the form of an upsetting, pointless rumination that fills the conscious attention to such extent that any other thought process can hardly take place.

2. At the tacit level, the activation of ambivalent, mixed feelings is matched, as a rule, by the surfacing of intrusive images of a bizarre nature and often having an almost hallucinatory vividness (Singer & Antrobus, 1972).

Because this excitation is not capable of a more adequate cognitive scaffolding, it will tend to be expressed through emotional outbursts in which a painful sense of uncontrollability is always intermingled with rituals and compulsive actions. There is usually some connection between the sensory quality of the intrusive images and feelings and the specific motor pattern and concrete meaning assumed by the rituals (e.g., tactile—dirt and washing). Lacking a cognitive mediation, the motor setting and autonomic activation that accompany the arousal of critical images and feelings will tend to be directly realized through actions leading to a perception that is opposite to the sensory quality in question.

The time course of an obsessive cognitive dysfunction, though vastly variable, shows a certain tendency toward stabilization. In other words, it is as though for many obsessives, striving for omniscience and total control, however aimlessly, was a more reassuring and economic device for attaining a sure, though negative, identity than reaching a sense of one's personal uniqueness based on the awareness of one's limitations and uncertainties would be. As a result, it rather frequently happens that what appears at first to be an existential crisis that may forshadow possible personal growth, becomes in actual fact a strongly disabling life condition, sometimes complicated by depressive or psychotic reactions.

The relation between obsession and depression has been highlighted more than once by clinical studies, although the nature of such a connection is still fundamentally unclear (Gittleson, 1966a, 1966b, 1966c). However, the fact that the obsessive developmental pathway shares with the depressive one the experience of uncontrollability (although in the former case it is the consequence of an excessively demanding environment, while in the latter it is the result of losses or separations) can perhaps explain the predisposition common to both organizations to exhibit intense reactions of helplessness in the face of perceived adversities.

Finally, since the basic concern of an obsessive P.C.Org. always revolves around the constant attempt to achieve a unitary, satisfactory identity, one can expect that in a small percentage of cases these attempts will produce true delusional reactions. Clinical studies indicate that an obsessive condition can change into a psychotic one in about 5% of cases (Black, 1974; Gittleson, 1966d).

CHAPTER ELEVEN

PRINCIPLES OF LIFESPAN DEVELOPMENTAL PSYCHOPATHOLOGY

The experiencing of time shows many peculiar features. . . . Among them, needless to say, one of the most striking seems to be this: the irreversibility of biological time. From inner subjective experience, as well as from external observation of living systems, it results that the time of living systems is a dimension oriented in a non-symmetric way. It flows in a one-way direction from birth on to development, maturation, reproduction, aging, and death. This unidirectionality regards not only human beings but also the whole of living systems evolved during millions of years. — Atlan (1979)

The aim of this concluding chapter is to draw a general outline of the patterns and processes that take place in the lifespan development of a P.C.Org. once it has acquired a stable structuring after adolescence and youth. However, because there are very few systematic studies on the evolving adult self, this chapter will ultimately be based, on conjecture—and assumptions and hypotheses will certainly prevail over presently available controlled data. In the first section, I shall attempt to illustrate the basic processes underlying the lifespan dynamic interplay between maintenance and change; while in the second, I shall dwell on the mechanisms regulating the discontinuous emergence of major life transitions. The last section will be dedicated to concluding considerations about the continuity and unitarity that can be observed in an individual lifespan trajectory.

DEVELOPMENT AS A LIFELONG, DIRECTIONAL PROCESS

Contrary to the assumptions of those who believe in the traditional biological growth approach to development, early adulthood does not coincide with any special state of maturity, nor can it be regarded as a sort of end product whose only function is to maintain as stable as possible the attained homeostatic equilibrium. Instead, transformations and changes take place throughout the entire course of life, although patterns and processes by which the orthogenetic progression of development unfolds are basically different from those of maturational stages (Baltes, 1979; Baltes, Reese, & Lipsitt, 1980; Brent, 1978a, 1984; Lerner & Busch-Rossnagel, 1981; Lerner et al., 1980; Werner, 1957).

According to the orthogenetic principle, the fundamental progression of lifespan development is defined by an overall increase in the order and complexity of a P.C.Org. as a result of ongoing assimilation of experience. While during the maturational stages of development, the unfolding of cognitive growth allows for the progressive integration of contingent and concrete nuclear scripts into more general and abstract metascripts, from early adulthood onward abstract/formal thought and the reflexive dimension of consciousness (self-awareness) connected to it permit an endless process of further differentiation and integration of such metascripts.

In other words, the individual's thematic content—stemming from the oscillative emotional polarities of meaning—maintains its prominence and continuity throughout adulthood. Furthermore, the increased order and complexity brings about continuous shifts in the thematic content, making some specific topics more salient and emotionally charged than others (Haviland, 1983; Malatesta & Clayton Culver, 1984; Stewart, 1980, 1982; Stewart & Healy, 1984). In this way, the systemic coherence relating to the organizational unity of the personal meaning processes inherent to a specific P.C.Org. supplies a preferential direction to the unfolding of its orthogenetic progression during lifespan development. Consequently, there is the possibility of identifying what could be the "ideal" or normative positive progression of each P.C.Org. previously described.

For a depressive-prone individual, the positive progression should be identified with a continuous differentiation and integration of the loss theme, until he/she perceives it as a category of human experience rather than as a personal destiny of loneliness and rejection. Vice versa, the ideal directionality of an eating disorder P.C.Org. should lead the subject to an ever-growing sense of his/ her individuality and uniqueness, regardless of ongoing relationships with significant others; whereas, in both phobic and obsessive P.C.Orgs., the positive progression should lead (by way of totally different patterns and processes) to a growing sense of one's personal worth based on the progressive acknowledgment and acceptance of one's emotional domain—and consequently, to an increased capacity to experience and understand, with minimal distress, the complexity and ambiguity peculiar to the human interpersonal domain.

As previously mentioned, these directionalities are simply ideal trajectories of adult development that can be subject, at any time, to distortions and regressive shifts, and are always extremely variable from one individual to the other. Therefore, they may be viewed in the same way as one would identify an ideal or normative course of maturational stages despite the wide range of normal or pathogenic developmental pathways that it can generate.

The orthogenetic progression specific to each P.C.Org., however, plays a crucial role in establishing the individual's unitary sense of continuity and change throughout his/her lifespan. Both processes underlying such progression (i.e., the increase of organizational unity and self-awareness) can simultaneously produce both an equilibrating and a disequilibrating effect on the individual's systemic coherence. Let us now examine more closely the mechanisms involved in this oscillative interdependence between continuity and change.

1. The ability to store and process information into more and more abstract categories of personal meaning implies a progressive increase in the individual's organizational complexity. The opponent trends of continuity and change stemming from this process can be summarily described as follows.

Continuity is connected to the stabilizing effect resulting from the self's growing ability to synthesize past and present experiences into a more complex, ordered, and unitary personal view (Nozick, 1981; Stewart & Healy, 1984).

In contrast, disequilibrium and pressures for change can be ascribed to the fact that each increase in organizational complexity produces incongruities (inherent to the tacit oscillative self-boundaries) that are more likely to be articulated into explicit models and, therefore, to become more evident and unbearable for the individual. The clearest example of this has been reported in the eating disorder P.C.Org., in which increased organizational complexity due to emerging abstract thought almost inevitably leads to a disappointment in a beloved attachment figure and influences to a large extent the subsequent juvenile reorganization.

2. The unfolding of the reflexive dimension of consciousness into more complex and ordered levels is, in turn, matched by the progressive emergence of more integrated patterns of self-awareness. This simultaneously produces both equilibrating and disequilibrating effects.

Continuity is related to the growing sense of foreknowledge of, and anticipation in facing, novel situations, due to the increasingly complex self-monitoring and comparison of one's ongoing emotional reactions to related reactions in the past (Stewart & Healy, 1984). The stabilizing effect derives, therefore, from the fact that any actual perceptual level of consciousness (i.e., "having an experience") is immediately ordered into the reflexive–integrative dimension of consciousness (i.e., "being aware of having an experience") through which the information processed at the perceptual level is integrated as a whole with past memories and current beliefs.

Alternatively, disequilibrium and pressures for change are due to the fact that reflexive awareness produces a structural gap in individual knowledge between the ongoing perception of self and reality and the whole integrative dimension that perception is simultaneously assuming. Consequently, discrepancies between actual and ideal self become evident. Furthermore, besides the possibility of making the discrepancies in selfhood processes more evident, the increase in self-awareness seems in itself able to lead to the progressive emergence of a pervasive sense of ambiguity—for a single experience can have simultaneous but quite different interpretations or meanings. As Nagel (1979) suggested, this perceived ambiguity—connected perhaps to the existential sense of absurdity that many poets and writers have so poignantly described—could be considered to be the result of the match between two inescapable viewpoints; while an ongoing perception of ourselves makes our actions, plans, and wishes immediately necessary and believable, in regarding our lives, we invariably also have an outside point of view from which that same necessity and credibility can appear to be groundless and questionable.

Finally, it should also be stated, that the experience of ambiguity is scaffolded differently and exerts dissimilar pressures depending on the personal meaning processes involved in its appraisal and processing. For example, in depressive-prone individuals, the ambiguity experience may confirm their feelings about loneliness and uselessness of efforts, while in the eating disorder-prone it may render more pervasive the blurred and wavering sense of self. In phobic-prone subjects, the experience may worsen the need for protection or freedom, and in obsessionals it may make the search for ultimate certainty even more problematic.

BIFURCATION POINTS IN LIFESPAN
DYNAMIC EQUILIBRIUM

The essential tension between maintenance and change exhibited by a P.C.Org. is reflected in the one specific lifespan developmental dynamic equilibrium that in a systems/process-oriented approach has been appropriately called "order through fluctuations." This means that the higher-order patterns that emerge are the result of fed-forward oscillations aimed at integrating the fluctuations or disequilibriums arising from ongoing assimilation of experience (Brent, 1978b; Jantsch, 1980; Jantsch & Waddington, 1976; Mahoney, 1982, in press; Nicolis & Prigogine, 1977; Prigogine, 1976; Riegel, 1979; Weimer, 1983).

> The most important feature of this model . . . is its postulation that each new level of structural organization is a synthesis of previously antithetical forces. Thus, the occurrence of internal conflicts between different aspects of an organized system is a fundamental impetus for the process of organic development itself. Thus, within this model tension, conflict, and stress among the constituents of a structure is not in itself indicative of a problem within that structure, but merely the sign of the ongoing process of organic development. (Brent, 1984, p. 163)

In other words, while a P.C.Org. tends at any time in its lifespan toward a static, final equilibrium, it never succeeds in achieving it, and as a consequence, stability is an ongoing oscillative process in which the dynamic balance between the opponent equilibrating and disequilibrating trends is attained by continuously displacing the equilibrium attained each time by the system. Within this generative, endless directionality, the orthogenetic progression of a P.C.Org. is not ot a linear type because changes, rather than the consequence of uniform, day-after-day cumulation, are the emerging effect of discontinuous crises. This procedure is commonly found in the development of complex systems; even in the evolution of science, for instance, periods of rapid change and reorganization of scientific paradigms alternate with periods of relative stability (Kuhn, 1970, 1977).

The threshold points for the emergence of higher-order patterns are called *"bifurcation points."* This is because in connection with these points, a P.C.Org. drives in the direction of a new level of personal meaning processes reorganization by means of wide and random fluctuations. Whenever individuals reach a bifurcation point, they enter a sort of "metastable state" in which an even slight disequilibrium may activate deep irreversible changes in their felt identity (Brent, 1984). The quality of individual awareness, in turn, dramatically influences the subsequent scaffolding of changes started by a metastable state. Particularly, it will ultimately determine whether they will take on the form of a progressive or a regressive shift in comparison to the individual's ideal or normative orthogenetic progression.

> Under appropriate conditions, these changes culminate in the emergence of a new, higher level of development. Under less ideal conditions, the result may be a classical "nervous breakdown"—that is, a breakdown in the individual's ability to function even at a previous level. (Brent, 1984, p. 174)

Any lifespan development has, therefore, an oscillating and discontinuously biphasic trend. While in times of stability, the fluctuations between the individual's opponent polarities of personal meaning are quite regular and even predictable, in times of changes, both the kind and intensity of fluctuations and the organizational level to which the individual is now heading become widely unpredictable.

> Between two bifurcation points, the system follows deterministic laws (such as those of chemical kinetics), but near the points of bifurcation it is the fluctuations which play an essential role in determining the branch that the system chooses. Such a point of view introduces the concept of "history" into the explanation of the state of the system. (Allen, 1981, p. 29, quoted by Weimer, 1983)

A historical perspective is, in fact, essential in approaching the lifespan of any P.C.Org. This is because the structure of dynamic equilibrium during a period of stability becomes fully comprehensible only if one knows the organizational level reached by the individual as he/she went through the previous bifurcation point.

Finally, a systems/historical approach also implies that primacy be attributed to personal meaning processes in the scaffolding of significant life experiences, rather than to the supposed specificity of some life events capable of eliciting adult crises per se. Indeed, each P.C.Org. contains, in the specificity of its recursive oscillation between self-boundaries, the "internal cause" of its own crises, and a life event becomes critical only because of the meaning that it assumes within that self-referent logic. The critical role that a life event can play clearly does not imply the need for a conscious elaboration of such meaning, because what may often occur—to use an expression pertaining to the language of complex systems theorists—is that "what appears as noise and nonsense to the observer of the conscious level is in fact meaningful messages from the unconscious level" (Serres, 1976, quoted by Atlan, 1981, p. 202). It is from this perspective that we shall go on to analyze the most common processes underlying the emergence of bifurcation points in lifespan development.

Critical Periods in Adult Lifespan

A critical period is a "chronological window" in which a specific rearrangement of a set of individual variables is able to produce an equally specific, irreversible transition to another level of personal reorganization, rather rapidly and with relatively small effort (Brent, 1984).

While the existence of such periods during maturational stages seems now definitely accepted, there is a certain tendency to over-look their existence in adulthood, or to regard them as mere effects of social and environmental conditions, as opposed to previous "bio-maturational" critical periods. On the contrary, the orthogenetic progression, through the increased organizational complexity and reflexive consciousness, can modify the established equilibrium in the subjective perception of time directedness and give rise to internal irreversible transformations in experiencing past and future. These are capable in themselves of pushing the individual toward a bifurcation point. According to Prigogine (1973), irreversibility should be understood as a symmetry-breaking process; that is, as a break in the time symmetry between past and future. Thus, the evolution of a time-bound complex system, becomes possible only through the discontinuous emergence of symmetry-breaking processes. Considering the human lifespan development in this perspective, it becomes possible to identify bifurcation points in the subjective experience of the temporal dimension that are very similar to Prigogine's symmetry-breaking processes.

Each lifespan starts out with an almost total temporal symmetry (i.e., an exclusive sense of the present that in infancy and childhood is given by the immediacy of the experience of self and reality). Only through the subsequent adolescent symmetry breaking does a growing distinction between past and future emerge. At the time of the existential discovery of one's self-identity, in youth, the past is perceived as being just begun, and the person feels he/she faces an unlimited future full of potentialities.

This sense of the future is replaced, as time goes by, by another more restricted one connected to the consciousness of death and, with the beginning of middle age, one starts to feel embodied in a limited, unrepeatable, and irreversible existence. Finally, in the course of middle and old age, the future is less and less perceived as a projection toward alternative possibilities, and the sense of one's life is primarily based on a past that occupies, by now, nearly all of one's lifespan.

Needless to say, any transformation in one's sense of existential time unfolds a new space–time dimension, and therefore starts substantial changes in one's sense of self and world. Thus, it is reasonable to suggest that the surfacing of a symmetry-breaking process roughly coincides with the emergence of an adult critical period. However, as compared to the greater uniformity in time and explanatory continuity of maturational critical periods, adulthood stages exhibit, even with the same character of invariant progression, greater flexibility and indeterminateness. There are at least two fundamental reasons for this.

In the first place, individual differences in the concreteness–abstractness dimension largely influence the quality in which one scaffolds the emerging transformation of a sense of existential time into personal emotional domains. Secondly, individual differences in self-awareness deeply influence the quality of reorganization undertaken during the critical period, and therefore the quality of the achieved final state. In other words, the continuity exhibited by the maturational stages in which orthogenetic progression is rigidly regulated by biological factors (unfolding of logical/cognitive abilities) and revealing the same characteristics in the majority of subjects, is replaced in adult development by a greater indeterminateness, as orthogenetic progression now becomes regulated mainly by psychological factors (qualitative patterns of self-awareness) that are variable from one person to the other.

Convergent evidence coming mostly from longitudinal studies on life histories and biographies has supplied descriptive accounts of the features of the adult self at different stages of life and has provided support for the existence of adult critical periods. These periods are viewed as normative crises that highlight, on the one hand, the individual's transformation in experiencing subjective time and, on the other, his/her growing awareness of the irreversibility of the lifespan (Gould, 1978; Levinson, 1978; Sheehy, 1976; Stewart & Healy, 1984; Vaillant, 1977). These critical periods—each of which has a distinctive character for the specific developmental tasks and life issues that distinguish it from all others—show an invariant progression in the course of an individual lifespan. Such progression can be summarily described as follows.

Adolescence and Early Adulthood

This period, which covers the period from about age 17 to 22, signals the beginning of adulthood and can be considered a bridge that joins the late maturational stage and the first adult critical period. The emergence of abstract thought and of the consequent awakening of self-awareness (decentering from reality and recentering on the self) has the effect of making youth the period when the emergent irreversible directness of time is first projected into cognitive–emotional processes, producing an existential discovery of the future as a new personal dimension capable of being planned for and manipulated.

The main issue of the adolescent resolution is the programming of a life plan centered on the resolution of specific developmental tasks, such as the achievement of a sense of self as autonomous agency (separation from native family) and the elaboration of a hypothesis about the nature of one's participation in the adult world. As a matter of fact, constant reformulation of such developmental tasks goes on throughout the entire lifespan. On the one hand, as Levinson (1978) pointed out, any person remains a son or daughter, brother or sister throughout the course of life and, therefore, only the quality of the relationship with the native family is continuously revised. On the other hand, the nature of one's participation in the world of others must be constantly updated and renegotiated in consideration of subsequently acquired experience. As a result, the characteristic problem of youth is that the subject, still lacking any personal experience as a reference point, must nevertheless make a *first* formulation of a life plan, which makes this period usually a turbulent and specially critical one, with possible relevant consequences on the psychopathological level.

It should be specified that the first formulation of a life plan does not necessarily require a detailed planning, because it simply concerns the identification of a set of coherent general intentions and goals that are open to further detailing and revisions for the rest of one's life. Obviously, by providing the individual with a specific directionality, this first formulation will necessarily influence the revisions brought about by subsequent adult critical periods. Moreover, despite the emotional distress involved in the formulation of a life plan, the individual is generally not entirely aware of it because "a life plan can have and refer to a property without showing or communicating this" (Nozick, 1981, p. 577). It is in consequence of this gap between the individual's conscious intentions and his/her effective actions that a whole range of discrepant life events is likely to occur. These, in turn, play a crucial role in the further articulation and revision of the selected directionality.

The Dynamics of P.C.Orgs.' Cognitive Dysfunctions in Adolescence and Early Adulthood. The essential aspect in a cognitive dysfunction at this time of life is youngsters' difficulty in giving themselves a coherent personal rearrangement and commitment from which they can derive a sense of security and competence in taking the first steps into adulthood. In this phase, this basically consists of establishing new affectional bonds outside of one's parents. As previously remarked (see Chapter 4), this is usually the result of a hampered cognitive–emotional separation from parents that undermines the sense of self as independent agency and therefore reduces considerably the possibilities of autonomous affective commitments. The systemic coherence of personal meaning processes determines the specificity of the clinical picture pertaining to each P.C.Org. described in previous chapters.

In the eating disorder P.C.Org., the emergence of a blurred sense of self is the crucial feature matching the problematic separation from the family (disappointment in a beloved parent). Eating disorders express an attempt to take a stand in the face of this unbearable, critical felt identity. Thus, Susan's (p. 159) anorexic reaction right after the disappointment in her father was a way of acquiring, through the perceived control of her biological drives, a sense of strength and efficiency with which she could oppose her pervasive feelings of personal ineffectiveness and emptiness. Brenda's first bulimic attacks (p. 159) at the time of the disappointment in her mother were the only way in which the passive attitude toward herself and reality allowed her to fill and appease, at least temporarily, her distressing feeling of personal emptiness.

A perceived threat to one's need for protection is the distinctive feature of the phobic reaction to the adolescent pressures for a greater emotional detachment from the family and for forming new affectional bonds. The limitation of motor autonomy and the fear of losing control that Shirley (p. 74) felt as she first fell in love were her way of forcing herself to spend most of the time in the only environment that gave her enough protection—the family—at least until the world of her contemporaries appeared less dangerous and hostile.

In the obsessive P.C.Org., the same problems are revealed in the form of disturbances that generally concern either the attempt to reach absolute certainty about the soundness and lastingness of one's feelings (see Derek, p. 73) or the equally absolute need to feel perfectly able to control one's sexual impulses (see Alison, p. 183).

In the depressive P.C.Org., the juvenile helplessness reactions are usually connected to the pervading sense of loneliness deriving from perceived difficulties in establishing affectional bonds, or from desertions that often follow the first attempts at relationships with the other sex.

At 18, Eric (see pp. 51, 126, 133) found himself engaged for a few weeks in an affective relationship with a young woman slightly older than himself. The initiative came from the woman, perhaps out of curiosity about his solitary, secretive attitude, and he had accepted it with surprise. But, after a short while, the woman again took the initiative of ending this relationship that since the beginning had seemed stagnant and uninteresting to her. Eric's depressive reaction was so intense and lasting that his father intervened, and sent him to a famous psychotherapist for over a year. During therapy Eric progressively realized that rather than being a victim of the girl's whims and capriciousness, he had himself caused the separation with his rooted sense of unlovableness. From the very beginning, loss had seemed to him to be the certain and unavoidable ending to that relationship. From this, Eric concluded that loneliness was apparently for him the most suitable life condition. As a consequence, he almost totally excluded the affective domain from his life plan, and concentrated all his effort on becoming a serious and competent journalist.

As can be noticed, the most outstanding consequence of a clinically disturbed adolescence is the elaboration of a rather rigid and scarcely articulated life plan that has greater probability of being questioned in later stages of adulthood.

The Age-30 Transition

Around midadulthood (from about age 28 to 32) the increased order and complexity of an individual's experience of self and reality promotes a further temporal symmetry-breaking process that deeply modifies the sense of the future.

In contrast to the view during youth and early adulthood, the future is no longer perceived as an unlimited dimension of possibilities that are sure to come true sooner or later, but instead undergoes a sharp reduction of potentiality and becomes more defined in a personal, unrepeatable way. In other words, the subject realizes that time is no longer limitless and he/she loses the "frenzy of immortality" that is the prerogative of youth. Death is no longer a philosophic, abstract possibility that concerns mankind as a whole, but undergoes a process of personalization by which it is experienced for the first time as the very disintegration of one's real self.

This perceived finitude presses on the subject the need for a revision of the life-plan formulation made during the previous period. The specific developmental tasks during this stage entail the need for a stronger and more defined affective and professional commitment, as well as the necessity to be more self-concerned.

This transition may take many forms, but it invariably involves appreciable changes in the individual's perception of self and the world. Many times the transition is a smooth one. This is usually when the revision of one's life plan has proved somehow satisfactory, and one's competence and worthiness has received sufficient confirmation. The subject can then proceed with little concern to what Levinson (1978) called the "settling down period". It is during this time that individuals actively try to lay the foundations for a more defined structuring of their lives through affectional choices (marriage, etc.) and professional choices (beginning of new activities, greater commitment in chosen career, etc.) that are in accordance with their conceptions. In other cases, a distressing transition may take place if the revision is unsatisfactory and has evoked a radical correction of the original life plan. In these circumstances, big life changes can occur, which the subject may experience as true leaps in the void. For example, Robert Musil at age 30 was a renowned physicist of the Stuttgart Polytechnic. He decided almost suddenly to become an obscure librarian, who would, in financial need, write novels and comedies that very few people would read while he was alive.

The Dynamics of P.C.Orgs.' Cognitive Dysfunctions in the Age-30 Transition. Whenever it becomes too difficult to adequately control—let alone revise—one's life plan, the onset of a full-fledged clinical disturbance becomes most likely. While features and functions of these disturbances vary according to the systemic coherence of the different P.C.Orgs. (and are therefore similar to those described in the previous stage), the onset mechanism of such patterns has a common base that can be related to the abrupt redimensioning or disconfirmation of the life hypothesis elaborated during the adolescent resolution. The processes leading to such conditions vary according to the way certain life events are scaffolded into particular patterns of meaning that are critical for the individual.

A mere delay of an expected advancement to editor in chief was enough to activate the intense depression that overcame Eric at the age of 31 and required further psychotherapy. The disappointment led him to believe that his efforts through all those years had been useless and that the objective of becoming a competent journalist was no doubt an illusion. He had now lost everything—affectional life (long-since put aside) and working life that now proved to be a failure.

Albert's phobic reaction (p. 118) between the age of 32 and 33 was the result of his confused realization that the adolescent dream of becoming a famous, world-traveling scientist had instead progressively trapped him inside a family that he felt stranger to and a research institution where he regarded himself as a mere employee. The incident in which he was trapped in the elevator simply activated the sense of change that had been pervading him and that his blind attitude to emotions had previously prevented him from focusing upon.

The turmoil produced by the disappointment in her father had inspired in Susan (pp. 157, 167) the sense that only by becoming an active, efficient, self-controlled woman would she be able to face possible disappointments in her future affectional life. The anorexic reaction that she went through at age 29 was activated by the realization that she had let herself become excessively involved in a relationship that had seemed nothing more than a flirtation, and the belief that she did not have the "willpower" to leave her partner.

By giving a religious emphasis to her life plan and conforming to the principle of experiencing *only* positive, unselfish emotions, Alison (pp. 173, 183) had finally solved the problems connected to the struggle to control sexual impulses. She had long considered the idea of becoming a nun, but after much rumination and doubt, she had decided that the image of wife and mother, totally dedicated and self-sacrificing to the good of her beloved ones, was more suitable to her. At age 29, however, soon after her first pregnancy, she experienced a crisis when she was unable to admit that taking care of a baby, besides being a joyous exercise of virtue and altruism, could also produce annoyance and irritation. The obsessive pattern that gradually developed reflected her attempt to reach a final, conclusive certainty on the positive or negative nature of her real self.

The Midlife Transition

With the beginning of midlife (from about age 40 to 46), another temporal symmetry-breaking process further modifies one's sense of the future. Once again one's life structure comes into question.

The future loses another large portion of its potentialities and is increasingly perceived as something that is, in fact, already present; in other words, the future comes to coincide more and more with the "hic et nunc," and everything the person deems still possible must be done now or never. This is related to the growing presence of death awareness and gives the individual the chance of verifying conclusively whether goals selected in the previous life-structuring period could be considered true possibilities or mere illusions. Suddenly life does not seem to provide the great surprises or changes that one imagined would occur. If, for instance, throughout the 30s one had had the idea of eventually becoming the president of the corporation one was working for, now, entering the 40s, one is clear-sightedly able to assess whether this chance is real or is only an old device of young people to give themselves importance. The sense of being embodied, without chance of escape, in a limited existence that has produced irreversible situations and events becomes now growingly pervasive, and, as a rule, results in a certain degree of emotional turmoil, more or less marked by a sense of not knowing where to turn, or of being stagnant and unable to move at all (Levinson, 1978).

The principal developmental task expressing this essential concern of midlife involves the attempt to reorganize one's life plan, so as to take into account the struggling modifications in the sense of self and reality that the individual is experiencing. But, since the future is perceived as "presentified," the attempt to reorder one's life structure is carried out mainly by reappraising the past. Subjects' interest in their past history generally brings them to consider that the aspects of self that have been neglected should more urgently find adequate expression in the ongoing reordering. This makes possible the occurrence of even more major changes in one's lifestyle, such as divorces; search for new affective commitments; drastic changes in occupation; return to past habits and emotional styles; discovery of artistic creativity, intellectual gifts, and so on.

Apart from the intensity of the emotional distress, the midlife transition must be regarded, in any case, as a moderate to severe personal crisis and is, in my opinion, one of the major turning points of lifespan development, together with adolescence and youth. Most striking is the fact that, despite the intensity of the experienced struggling feelings, the majority of individuals are not fully aware of the transition they are going through. This often makes vainly wishful and fruitless the attempts to reorganize and further stabilize their emotional turmoil. At a time like this, an onset of clinical manifestations or a greater stabilization of past regressive shifts is likely to take place.

Robert Musil, the great Austrian writer so deeply interested in psychology and human feelings, left us an admirable description of the profound agitation that Ulrich, the main character in the novel *The Man Without Qualities*, felt on the threshold of midlife:

At this moment he wished to be a man without qualities. But this is probably not so very different from what other people sometimes feel too. After all, by the time they have reached the middle of their life's journey few people remember how they have managed to arrive to themselves, at their amusements, their point of view, their wife, character, occupation and successes, but they cannot help feeling that not much is likely to change any more. It might even be asserted that they have been cheated, for one can nowhere discover any sufficient reason for everything's having come about as it has. It might just as well have turned out differently. The events of people's life have, after all, only to the last degree originated in them, having generally depended on all sorts of circumstances such as the moods, the life or death of quite different people, and have, as it were, only at the given point of time come hurrying towards them. For in youth life still lies before them as an inexhaustible morning, spread out all round them full of everything and nothing; and yet when noon comes there is all at once something there that may justly claim to be their life now, which is, all in all, just as surprising as if one day suddenly there were a man sitting there before one, with whom one had been corresponding for twenty years without knowing him, and all the time imagining him quite different. But what is still much more queerer is that most people do not notice this at all; they adopt the man who has come to stay with them, whose life has merged with their own lives and whose experiences now seem to them the expression of their own qualities, his destiny their own merit or misfortune. Something has had its way with them like a fly-paper with a fly; it has caught them fast, here catching a little hair, there hampering their movements and has gradually enveloped them, until they lie buried under a thick coating that has only the remotest resemblance to their original shape. And then they only dimly remember their youth when there was something like a force of resistance in them. (1979, rev. ed., pp. 151–152)

The trend of the second half of life and the period of aging will depend largely on the way the individual has gone through the midlife turmoil, and especially on whether the reorganization has been carried out—to use Sheehy's (1976) terms—in the direction of renewal (with the structuring of a more authentic life structure) or of resignation (with the sense of staleness progressively stiffening in a defined and conflictual acquiescence). In the former case, the second portion of life can come to represent the best years of a lifespan, whereas, in the latter, the aging just begun is going to be a grudging, irritable one, full of regrets and claims about a possible better past that the hostility of the world has inexorably prevented.

The Dynamics of P.C.Orgs.' Cognitive Dysfunctions in the Midlife Transition. When a poor articulation of the concreteness–abstractness dimension has led a P.C.Org. to complete the previous adult transitions with precarious or distorted reorganizations, it is much more likely that the midlife transition will lead to a sort of "resignation resolution" characterized by a stabilization and acceptance of one's sense of staleness and inability to structure a more effective attitude toward life.

Emotional disorders, either appearing for the first time or representing a stabilization of the ones that emerged before, will tend to progressively assume the characteristics of a true lifestyle. In other words they will be directed at scaffolding the perceived restriction and limitation of one's possibilities into a specific life structure according to the personal meaning processes underlying the systemic coherence of every P.C.Org.

At the age of 41, Albert, after having adequately managed the phobic reaction experienced at age 32–33, slowly fell in a state of apathy, indolence, and indifference. In the same period, position changes in his research institution had cut him off completely from attaining a post that he always hoped for, that of director of a specific section.

One night, as he was watching TV, he suffered a panic attack and intense tachycardia. In the course of the following 2 weeks, he had two more attacks. As opposed to what had happened 8 or 9 years earlier, these episodes did not produce an acute onset of a phobic reaction, but rather a very selective anxious focusing on every possible bodily reaction, so much so that within a short period of time he could no longer work. A number of strange feelings kept him in constant fear, and he could only feel relieved when he went to doctors or was reassured by people he trusted or by repeatedly consulting medical textbooks.

After 2 or 3 months, perhaps reassured by all the checkups that positively excluded any organic disease, Albert felt he could better control the state of alarm that still persisted, though to a lesser degree. Thus, he cautiously went back to work. However, at work, his attention was extremely focused on his body and on a whole series of diseases that he seemed always on the point of coming down with. As a result, he gradually reduced his social activities and avoided nearly every working engagement, so that, almost without realizing it, he was gradually pushed aside in the institution. In other words, because of the establishment of the typical vicious circle by which an emotional distress produces irreversible choices at the professional and social levels that, in turn, confirm and further develop the same emotional distress, Albert's limiting situation was subject to progressive stabilization within 3–4 years.

Giving up all effort to stay on a diet and accepting obesity as a stable self-image was Brenda's (pp. 60, 62, 75, 159, 168) way of building a life structure consistent with an internal causal attribution that made her experience affectional disappointments throughout her life (now concluding with the final breakup of her marriage) as due to the unacceptability of her body image.

Taking the cases of Albert and Brenda as typical of midlife cognitive dysfunctions, I may end by stating that the earlier adult clinical disorders show, in the course of a lifespan, a tendency to undergo progressive unification and stabilization, and often mingle with troubles typical of old age. Although extensive and controlled longitudinal research is not yet available, several preliminary studies seem to encourage this supposition. To quote an example, Adam (1982) in an attachment theory perspective, remarked that in the lifespan of depressive-prone individuals there is a characteristic shifting from suicide attempts in early adulthood toward actual suicides in later life:

> The peaking of suicide attempts in the earlier adult years could be seen as a manifestation of more active attachment behaviors among a group prone to form insecure attachments but with abundant opportunities for them, whereas the increase in actual suicide in later life may reflect the greater vulnerability to the consequences of loss that is associated with the diminished opportunity to form new relationships. (p. 290)

THE NOTION OF LIFE THEME

What ruins us, what always has ruined us, is our longing for a destiny, *any* kind of destiny.—Cioran (1979)

In the course of life, each individual will find him/herself proceeding along a unique and irreversible developmental pathway whose trajectory is, in turn, the ongoing dynamic product resulting, on the one hand, from the ideal or normative directionality stemming from the individual's systemic coherence and, on the other hand, from his/her integrative ability to articulate it throughout adulthood transitions and significant life events.

The irreversibility of a life history depends on the ongoing transformation of subjective time brought about by the individual and is expressed by a progressive and coherent integration between the subject's past and actual self stages. This memory-unifying process progressively decreases the opportunities that the individual has—as a "self-justifying historian" (Greenwald, 1980)—to revise and modify his/her past history. Nozick (1981) has developed this point quite poignantly:

> The self synthesizes itself not only transversely, among things existing only at that time, but also longitudinally so as to include past entities, including past selves which were synthesized. My currently synthesized self includes past stages in accordance with a closest continuer and a closest predecessor schema. Will the self continually rewrite its history, like a Soviet historian disowning and rewriting a currently undesired past? There are limits on this; when some past self-stage is incorporated in a synthesis, brought in also is its conception of its past, as incorporated in its own self-synthesis. And while one may attribute a mistake to one's past self about its past self, this will not be done casually—the mistake would have to be explained. Thus, generally, my past self's past will be carried into the current synthesizing as my own, too. (p. 91)

These limits to one's information-processing capacity—which, as suggested by Pribram (1980a), rather than reflecting a sort of fixed capacity of the brain for processing information, are due to the *pattern* with which information has been organized—make the regulatory function exerted by personal identity and attitude toward oneself increase in the course of the lifespan. That is, during juvenile and early adult stages, even a consistent transformation of one's felt identity is possible, but as the person goes on in middle and late adulthood the possibilities of a significant identity change gradually decrease.

> In short, the coherent, differentiated self of adulthood acts as a brake on personality change, and provides for constructed, reflected continuity. It does not, and could not, preclude change, for the equilibrium of the self can be threatened, yielding a new process of differentiation,

abstraction, and integration. But if the self is integrated on a base of rich differentiation and many-layered abstractions, revolutions in the self in adulthood will probably be rare (especially if the differentiation and abstractions in turn derive from a broad base in affective experience). (Stewart & Healy, 1984, p. 285)

As Luckmann (1979) pointed out, personal identity tends to become a historical form of life and the progressive merging and integration in the individual memory of both past and actual self-stages leads, on the one side, to an even greater intertwining between the lifestyle and the image of self and, on the other, to a growing "rigidity" of the lifestyle, with a consequent gradual decrease of perceived alternatives. Indeed, terms such as "plan of life" (Nozick, 1981; Popper & Eccles, 1977), or "life theme" (Csikszentmihalyi & Beattie, 1979) have been used to indicate the individual lifespan tendency toward unification and undirectionality that appears with striking clarity each time. In a biography, we have the impression that the character in question has moved, without even knowing it, along a "guiding track" or, to use theater terminology, has followed a "script."

Needless to say, in a systems/process-oriented approach, a life theme is something dynamically constructed day by day and year by year. It is based upon the events by which the individual has scaffolded his/her life transitions, the way he/she has interpreted and dealt with them, and of the consequences of this process. The results of these choices and actions, in turn, become events to be further synthesized in an even more comprehensive image of self and the world, revealing to the individual with growing clearness how compulsory and unrepeatable is the trajectory of his/her past life.

CONCLUDING REMARKS

The notion of P.C.Org. has been the base on which both the theoretical framework and the derivative tentative model of psychopathology rest. Having come to the end of the present work, I would like to devote a few paragraphs to summarizing what has been presented and to offer some concluding explanatory notes.

1. According to this perspective, human beings may be regarded as complex, historical knowing systems that in the process of scaffolding reality into assimilable sequences of experience exhibit a tendency to structure certain invariant self-recursive ordering patterns in the articulation of their personal meaning processes. However, I wish to stress the fact that each of the P.C.Orgs. described in previous chapters is not intended to represent an "entity," made up of specific knowledge contents, but rather is a *unitary ordering process*, capable of scaffolding a wide variety of possible knowledge contents according to a basic invariant personal meaning structure. For instance, consider an event of a general nature such as bereavement. Although characterized by an informational content that is more or less the same for everybody (loss of a significant person), the quality of the grief process with which the bereavement is assimilated will vary according to the P.C.Org. involved. For a depressive the processing will take the form of loneliness and a feeling that life is useless; a phobic will feel threatened in his/her need for protection; an eating disorder-prone person will develop an even more blurred and wavering sense of self; and an obsessive will try to attain ultimate, final certainty about personal, moral, and social responsibilities that preceded and accompanied the event. In other words, the organizational unity of personal meaning processes defines the kind of systemic coherence to which a P.C.Org. is constrained during its lifespan development and consequently biases the way significant events and life transitions are assimilated.

2. Because human development is a complex, multilinear progression characterized by the embeddedness of its patterns and processes, each individual may be regarded as a unique experiment of nature. As a result, it is very unlikely to find in reality an absolutely "pure" P.C.Org. For example, consider the depressive P.C.Org. It may very well happen that a person suffers the loss of one parent in childhood and, at the same time, is restrained in exploratory behavior by the other parent. In this case, the grounds for both depressive and agoraphobic developmental pathways are simultaneously laid. Using the same line of reasoning, a depressive developmental pathway can combine with obsessive or eating disorders pathways, and the same can be said of any other P.C.Org.

Although as a general rule different components are present in tacit self-boundaries, the organizational unity of the emotional domain makes *one specific pattern of organizational closure prevail hierarchically over others*, lending unitarity and coherence to the individual personal meaning processes. A clinical vignette is no doubt the best exemplification of this aspect.

The attachment patterns of affectionless control that marked Eric's maturational stages (pp. 51, 126, 133, 198), besides giving him a sense of affectional loss and incompetence, had also strongly reduced his exploratory behavior. Eric's typically depressive, compulsive, self-reliant attitude was intermingled with an extreme sensitivity in perceiving most affectional bonds as constrictive. Therefore in the course of his life he had avoided such forms of affectional stability as living together, fatherhood, and so on.

Around the age of 40, he underwent a considerable personal revolution, for which he sought therapeutic help and advice. He was directed to me by several colleagues and from the start he showed the firm intention of revising all his past life choices, to the point that—without any pressure on my part—he soon married and accepted the idea of possible fatherhood. A few months later, during a session, he announced that he and his wife were expecting their first child. Seeing that he was rather depressed in a circumstance that usually causes at least some enthusiasm, I asked him how he was experiencing these first steps on the way to fatherhood. After some thinking, he responded that he felt it as an intolerable burden and constriction, because it could only mean for him an irreversible limitation of his personal freedom. Surprised by what seemed, apparently, a typical phobic answer, I then asked what he meant by personal freedom. Eric's reply was a brilliant example of how the oversensitivity to constrictions produced by developmental interferences in exploratory behavior can be decodable only through the prevailing central meaning structures represented by loss: "To feel free has always meant for me that I can kill myself whenever I choose to. You can well understand that now, with this responsibility of a small child, I can no longer do that. Life has succeeded in trapping me, once and for all."

The patterns of organizational closure that differentiate personal meaning processes should therefore be considered as essentially conceptual devices that permit the gathering of data and the formulation of problems in a systemic fashion, that is, as sort of "clues" to identity forms of spontaneous personal organizations that configurate inside a complex domain such as the human self-conscious mind.

3. Finally, in a systems perspective, normalcy, neurosis, and psychosis—rather than static, fixed entities—should be seen as dynamic, changeable states of a P.C.Org's. systemic coherence, whose borders are indistinct most of the time. Consequently, along the normalcy–psychosis continuum, normalcy comes to correspond to the flexibility and generativity with which a P.C.Org. articulates its fundamental orthogenetic progression throughout its lifespan, as well as to the higher levels of organized complexity and self-transcendence that it is consequently able to achieve. On the other hand, the same P.C.Org., depending on the quality and elaboration of developmental experiences, can evolve toward a "neurotic" condition if the concreteness–abstractness dimension is insufficiently articulated, or slide to a "psychotic" condition if, in addition to the limit represented by a too concrete processing, there is also an interference in the self-synthesizing ability that provides functional unity to personal identity. In other words, neurosis and psychosis are nothing but different "languages"—expressed by different but parallel states of individual consciousness—that the same pattern of organizational closure can assume as a function of the individual's self-synthesizing ability.

I am, of course, well aware that the arguments and hypotheses expressed in this book are open to many criticisms from the point of view of scientific accuracy in data collecting, ordering, and comparison. However, the search for an explanatory—rather than merely descriptive—model of human knowledge and consciousness is not currently sustained by an adequate experimental methodology in psychological inquiry.

Consistent with the empiricist approach that reduced the study of psychology to the description of the interaction between organism and environment, experimentation thus far has been too fragmented, too focused on the isolation of details, and it has sometimes given the impression of being persued as an end in itself. In continuing to isolate and study single variables, moreover, psychologists tacitly endorse the view that there is an external ordered reality that can be discovered through a gradual and "objective" approach. Their strategy is to pose discrete and definite questions and wait for reality to supply clear and "factual" answers. What is striking in this attitude is the lack of integration and the scarcity of hypotheses as compared to the experimental methods, which are generally more complex and sophisticated. It is as though psychologists, instead of using experiments to check their hypotheses, were employing experimentation in the place of hypotheses. Thus, in spite of an abundance of studies on limited aspects of attitudes, cognitive abilities, or emotional processing, both in normal and abnormal psychology, there is an almost total lack of explanatory hypotheses of some complexity and consistency capable of directing the search for possible correlations between these sets of isolated data.

Under these conditions, it is clearly quite difficult to recognize that the same reality we regard as objective is constantly transformed by our self-conscious mind. In particular, the individual's "psychological dimension" has by now become a basic constituent of our culture, determining to a large extent the very forms that experience assumes. As a result, a whole set of phenomena known as "anxiety," "neurosis," and so on, virtually unknown to previous epochs, have acquired all those attributes that define them as "real." The fact is that no other epoch has ever experienced such self-consciousness as characterizes the present one. As expressed by Cioran (1956), from this viewpoint, the Renaissance is barbaric, the Middle Ages are mere prehistory, and even the 19th century can appear a little childish.

What are the effects of increased self-consciousness on the human way of experiencing and structuring reality, particularly on psychological welfare? The basic problem is that, lacking an explanatory theory of the mind, we are in no position to assess what kind of correlation exists between an increased self-consciousness and a perception of ambiguity that seems to go with it. Thus we still do not grasp the mechanisms underlying the emergence and dynamics of complex, disequilibrating emotions such as boredom, sense of absurdity, and so on, that increasingly pervade whole aspects of our culture and everyday life. On the one hand, we witness a proliferation of identity crises, on the other, because of the doubts we still have about the scientific nature of the self, we lack the ability to understand and face them. In a way, one of the most ironic paradoxes of contemporary psychology consists of wondering whether the self really exists in a world made unlivable by self-consciousness.

The search for a more comprehensive explanatory model of selfhood processes seems to me the only way that can lead us to elaborate future psychotherapeutic models capable of providing plausible answers to modern man's crises. For this reason, and in spite of the many limits that presently restrain this search for an explanatory model, I believe this should be our purpose. The present work can be better understood if seen mainly as an attempt in this direction.

SOME STRATEGIC PRINCIPLES FOR COGNITIVE THERAPY

Is there such a thing as the knowledge of men? We shall
remember, from time to time, that understanding a man is
nothing but reacting psychically to him in a well determined
manner. —Musil

A human knowing system reflects a dynamic equilibrium unfolding through successively more integrated models of self and the world. As will be elaborated below, this perspective has some remarkable consequences for the therapeutic approach.

In the usual cognitive–behavioral approaches, based on the rather static conception of a circular equilibrium regulated only by feedback mechanisms, therapy essentially aims at restoring the lost equilibrium, by increasing self-control and providing more practical problem-solving procedures. In contrast, the basic question on which a systems/process-oriented approach to cognitive therapy revolves can be formulated in this way: How can clients be aided in their personal temporal becoming to assimilate the disequilibriums that have thus far thwarted their attempts to reach more integrated levels of knowledge and self-awareness? In the discussion that follows, I shall attempt to elaborate the possible relevance of this shifting of basic questions for clinical and therapeutic pursuits.

THE "TRUTH PROBLEM" AND THE THERAPIST'S ATTITUDE TOWARD THE THERAPEUTIC RELATIONSHIP

To begin with, the cognitive analysis does not focus on the relationships between single beliefs or specimens of internal dialogue and some defined external stimulus. On the contrary, a systemic cognitive analysis is more comprehensive and revolves around two basic questions.

1. What kind of developmental stages brought about this individual P.C.Org.?
2. In what way is that P.C.Org. determining the very form of moment-to-moment experience?

Focusing on these questions, it becomes possible to delineate the basic assumptions about self and the world upon which the individual's very sense of reality rests. This, in turn, affords the therapist a better understanding of some of the crucial problems that emerge in any treatment. Why are some past experiences, although present in individual memory, completely neglected? Why are new experiences during therapy so difficult to assimilate in spite of their evident logical consistency?

To put it another way, the so-called truth problem is a fundamental question for both theoretical and clinical psychology. Indeed, it is well known that any epistemology presupposes—often implicitly—metaphysical assumptions about the basic question arising from human interaction with the world, such as, "what is the truth?" and "how can the truth be detected?"

In the empiricist–associationistic approach, the problem was solved by regarding truth as a copy of external reality having direct correspondence with it. Thus conceived, truth was considered singular, static, and external to man; all other possible views of the world were understandable only when compared to it. Consequently, the therapist's task was to evaluate the rationality–irrationality of clients' thoughts and beliefs according to external standards taken for true. Therapies conducted from such a perspective very often become pedagogical, intentionally seeking—and even creating—any useful opportunity to show the client his/her irrationality (e.g., see some techniques of Rational–Emotive Therapy; Ellis, 1962).

Viewing the problem from a different perspective, it is the individual's P.C.Org. itself that, in order to make reality "real," must possess a concept of truth or, if you prefer, something that plays the same logical role. Briefly, a systems approach regards truth as stemming from the core of an individual P.C.Org. and therefore as something belonging uniquely to each individual. Each person, through his/her tacit, basic assumptions, orders his/her conscious representations of self and the world and becomes capable of making a rather stable and reliable demarcations between what he/she considers real and unreal. Psychotherapy based on such a perspective does not aim at persuading clients to adopt other standards for truth, but rather at helping them to recognize, understand, and better conceptualize their own personal truth—this being their only possibility for making reality real.

Needless to say, a perspective of this kind implies a dramatic change in current conceptions on rationality. Rationality, rather than being something static and absolute like an entity, has a relativistic and interactive nature. In the first place, it is a basic process inherent to any human knowing system, and second, this process unfolds into knowledge structures only through the scaffolding of experience that takes place during individual temporal becoming. Moreover, since it stems from the core of an individual P.C.Org., rationality can by no means be considered only something belonging to the realm of formal logic or deductive, analytical thinking; on the contrary, it includes tacit schemata and emotional aspects that have been traditionally regarded as dogmatic, that is, irrational or, at least, not rational. From this viewpoint, therefore, the whole set of tacit assumptions and explicit thought procedures that give internal coherence and reliability to an individual P.C.Org. are considered rational for that specific individual, regardless of their correspondence to the classic norms of logic.

At a clinical level, a therapeutic approach based on this perspective considerably changes the structure of the therapeutic relationship as well as the strategy for facilitating a cognitive change. Rather than a pedagogic approach, therapy becomes an exploratory collaboration enabling the client to identify the basic assumptions that underlie his/her way of experiencing reality that have to be modified not because they are irrational but because they represent an outmoded solution. They were useful when first developed, but now, in a changed environment, they have fostered a world representation with little understanding power and repetitious, stereotyped, problem-solving strategies. Likewise, the therapeutic intervention is not considered a set of techniques designed to persuade the client to accept more "rational" points of view, but rather a strategy to modify the client's demarcation between real and not-real and to allow him/her to assimilate (e.g., to consider now as real) neglected past memories and new available experiences.

ASSESSMENT AND THE ROLE OF DEVELOPMENTAL ANALYSIS

In a therapeutic situation, the assessment procedure is a technical way of building up explicit, conceptual models to make underlying tacit processes evident and act on them.

At the beginning, the therapist can catch a glimpse of the quality of crucial tacit rules involved in the clinical picture through a careful behavioral and cognitive analysis of clients' causal theories about their complaints. Although the client's causal theories are not directly informing us about his/her actual ongoing processes (Nisbett & Wilson, 1977), they are nevertheless influenced by the same tacit rules, and so are useful as indirect information about them.

The assessment can be aided by providing clients with rationales for, and methods of, self-observation. As their observational and analytic skills improve, clients acquire the ability to distance and decenter themselves from certain engrained beliefs and self-images that were considered unquestionable, allowing the deeper structures underlying their conceptions of self and the world to emerge. Moreover, in the assessment procedure, the therapist should not let the emotional level go unnoticed while focusing only on the conscious cognitive processes immediately available. On the contrary, one has to work actively on emotional aspects, being careful from the start that every explanation assimilated by the client is paralleled by a coherent emotional labeling. In other words, one has to be constantly testing the labeling of emotions that accompany understanding processes. In such way a therapist can, on the one side, acquire data about the subject's personal range of recognizable emotions and, on the other, have the opportunity to supply explanations about the nature and functions of emotions and their labeling.

By now the therapist has a draft of the client's cognitive models that would allow him/her to render a reconstruction of the tacit rules underlying the client's maladaptive behavior. However, he/she cannot afford to indulge in groundless hypothetical reconstructions no matter how original and stimulating they might be. As a next step, a careful developmental analysis is carried out that provides the necessary frame of reference for the therapist to reconstruct the interplay between distressing events and cognitive processing abilities that step-by-step have led to the maintenance of a specific self-identity and attitude toward reality.

It should be made clear, however, that while the therapist is reconstructing the history of a client's development, he/she should not be limited to the events in themselves, but should consider that the particular effects of a stressful event are largely dependent on previous history and on cognitive abilities at that stage. The eating disorders provide a clear example. It seems quiet evident that both obesity and anorexia have their starting point in a similar stressful event, that is, a strong disappointment from a loved person, usually a parent. The different effects resulting from the same event have to be attributed to the different developmental stage at which that event occurred. In obese clients, the disappointment was experienced in childhood; cognitive abilities available at that time were not capable of coping with the event, making the subject experience it as an overwhelming failure. In anorexic clients, the disappointment occurred in adolescence, when emerging higher cognitive abilities were capable of coping with the event more or less effectively, making the subject experience it as an unbearable challenge to be striven against.

Once the developmental history has been reconstructed, the therapist is usually able to achieve three basic tasks: (1) step-by-step reconstruction of the client's cognitive models of self and reality and corresponding patterns of attitude toward him/herself; that is, the client's P.C.Org. and the current discrepancy between existing range of stability and deep oscillations to be assimilated; (2) identification of the client's tacit assumptions and thought procedures influencing their scaffolding of the experiential domain in which disequilibrium was produced; (3) assessment of the particular historical stage of the individual lifespan in which the disequilibrium occurred.

At this point, it becomes generally possible to provide clients with a better understanding of how they have organized their experience and, at the same time, to elaborate a therapeutic strategy in keeping with that understanding.

As a conclusion it is useful to bear in mind that the assessment procedure is just a reconstruction of tacit rules and by no means a one-to-one translation of them. The great epistemologist Lakatos used to say to his students that since men are not altogether rational, real history is less rational than its reconstruction.

THE MODELING OF THE THERAPEUTIC RELATIONSHIP AND CLIENTS' RESISTANCE TO CHANGE

Knowing the basic elements of the P.C.Org. that underlie the pattern of disturbed behavior and emotions, the therapist can behave, from the beginning, in such a way as to build a relationship as effective as possible for that particular client. In other words, the therapist should be able to establish a relationship that respects the client's personal identity and systemic coherence and that, at the same time, does not confirm the basic pathogenic assumptions. For example, in working with agoraphobics, the therapist has to respect their self-images centered on the need to be in control. He/she can do this by avoiding any direct attack on their controlling attitudes and by leaving them a wide margin of control in the relationship. At the same time the therapist should avoid confirming their assumptions about the somatic origin of their emotional disturbances or about their inborn fragility. In short, the therapist who can anticipate the models of self and reality tacitly entertained by the client is surely better able to help the development of a cooperative and secure therapeutic relationship than the therapist who cannot make such anticipations.

However, even though the modeling of the therapeutic relationship according to the client's P.C.Org. generally reduces resistances, they still emerge during therapy, being perhaps the expression of the same oscillative aspects that open complex systems exhibit in their evolving. More specifically, in the category of resistances to change found frequently in therapeutic practice are included phenomena such as those discussed by Liotti (1984).

1. More or less explicit objections raised by clients to therapist's prescriptions and explanations.

2. Relapses following the attainment of desired changes.
3. Report of expected difficulties in some significant interpersonal relationship (including the relationship with the therapist) as a consequence of the application of therapeutic principles.

Instead of striving directly to overcome these resistances, a process-oriented therapist tries to make use of them in order to assess the client's "theories" that have been challenged by the use of the therapeutic strategy (Bugental, 1978; Bugental & Bugental, 1984). In other words, resistances are an expression of the systemic coherence exhibited by the client's P.C.Org. and should therefore be considered, sources of meaningful information that may be used as a lead to uncover specific aspects of the client's developmental history. Moreover, the discussion of these aspects may help the client accept the novelty implied by the foreseen change without having too strong and frightening feelings that the change will imply a radical and abrupt modification of perceived personal identity.

I also wish to point out that the therapeutic relationship is an essential variable in all psychotherapy, and, in particular, that the client's positive involvement in the relationship is undoubtedly a facilitating factor in achieving the therapy's objectives. Presently, however, we are still far from having reached an exhaustive model of the interdependence between affect and cognition, and therefore we know little about the mechanisms underlying the way in which interpersonal relationships facilitate knowledge assimilation and change processes. Unfortunately, because of this state of affairs, the therapist's ability to use relationship dynamics to facilitate change is still mainly an art rather than a science. Bowlby's (1977b) approach to the therapeutic relationship in terms of attachment theory is presently one of the most promising hypotheses for the study of possible correlations between emotional aspects of the therapeutic relationship and therapeutic change.

SUPERFICIAL AND DEEP CHANGE

Two levels of therapeutic modification in cognitive psychotherapy can be identified: a superficial change and a deep change (Arnkoff, 1980; Mahoney, 1980).

A superficial change coincides with the reorganization of the client's attitude toward reality without revising his/her personal identity. This level of modification in many cases allows a real improvement in the client's adaptation to the environment and a reduction of emotional distress.

On the other hand, deep change involves a reorganization of the patterns of attitude toward oneself—giving individual consciousness an access to new sets of tacit, meaningful information on the self—and gradually leads to a restructuring of the client's perceived personal identity. Greenberg (1984) was able to experimentally demonstrate that the resolution of intrapersonal conflicts in a successful psychotherapy involves a deeper experiencing and appreciation of aspects of self that, though extremely affect-laden, had been neglected up to that moment.

These two types of change do not exclude one another; but, according to clinical experience, it is often possible to reach a deep change only through a preceding superficial one. However the request for a deeper analysis and change has to come from clients, while the therapist should only stimulate their curiosity. There are two essential reasons for this: First, deep analysis, as a process, is always accompanied by intense, often painful, emotions that the client should not be forced to undergo. Second, a "real" personal change can occur only if clients are enabled to produce it by themselves, which requires their complete willingness.

When the client asks for a deeper change, it is useful to work again on the developmental history, asking the client to participate as much as possible. Generally at this point the subject already knows his/her developmental history, because it was already used for obtaining a superficial change. Now it becomes possible to regard the past history from a different angle. In simpler terms, the therapist's basic question could be the following: "Okay, as we know, you have elaborated this conception of yourself through your past history. Well, in order to understand the degree of consistency and functionality of your self-image, we have to re-examine your history and recognize the whole set of "proofs" and "confirmations" that you have considered as supporting the theories about yourself throughout development. After that, we can examine the epistemological validity of such proofs and confirmations."

In a way, using such procedures, the therapist is able to work on the client's memory (Bara, 1984), leading him/her to focus on the differences between episodic contingent memories and the global meanings attributed to them. By way of such patient, accurate work, a progressive restructuring of personal meaning processes is possible, that is matched by a reordering of affect-laden events and scenes that takes place in the subject's memory. In turn, this therapeutic achievement becomes a further starting point for a quite stable reordering of the client's perceived personal identity.

THE STRATEGY FOR THERAPEUTIC CHANGE

Let us assume that the therapist is now directly facing the problem of guiding a client to assimilate the disequilibrium that thwarted prior attempts to reach more integrated level of knowledge. An assimilation of this kind generally becomes possible only through a revision of the cognitive models of self and reality entertained by clients.

In a personal letter, Bowlby (July 1982) suggested the following steps to achieve such a revision:

> For anyone to revise a cognitive model is, as you well know, a difficult undertaking. Principal tasks of the therapist I believe to be: (a) encouraging and enabling the patient to explore his cognitive models; (b) helping the patient to recognize the cognitive models he is actually utilizing; (c) helping him trace how he has come to have them, which I believe to have been in large measure due to his having accepted what his parents have constantly *told* him—both about themselves and about himself; (d) encouraging him to review the models in the light both of their history and also of the degree to which they correspond to his own *first-hand* experience of himself and his parents; (e) helping him recognize the sanctions his parents have used to insist that he adopts their model and not his own. Only after this process has been gone through many times are the revised models likely to be stable.

I fully subscribe to these ideas of Bowlby's and I would like to indicate some of the convergent aspects inherent in our respective clinical perspectives.

In a systems/process-oriented perspective, the possibility of reaching more integrated and comprehensive models of self and reality are strictly dependent on the individual's ability to make explicit the available sets of tacit rules. So, while proceeding along the steps proposed by Bowlby, the therapist's fundamental aim is to enable clients to consciously elaborate alternative representative models capable of better recognizing and structuring the tacit processes that are already influencing their thought procedures, albeit outside their sphere of awareness.

This notion has certain consequences on the attitude the therapist will assume in the therapeutic situation. That is, a therapist should bear in mind that the knowledge content capable of revising the client's cognitive models is already available in some way. What is not available is the client's selective attention in recognizing it. Thus, the therapist should pay great respect to the client's self-knowledge. In general, it is useless and even dangerous to put new knowledge into the client's head in any possible way, since the information useful to the client comes from his/her deep structures and cannot be replaced by the therapist's conceptions about life.

In such a perspective, therefore, it might be possible to revise our conceptions concerning directiveness versus nondirectiveness. They could be seen as complementary aspects rather than opposite ones. In order to make the tacit explicit, one has to directly encourage the client to elaborate a more integrated view of him/herself, but in order to do this, one has to respect the client's tacit level since it represents the essential directionality to be followed. For example, it is useless and dangerous to try to convince individuals with depressive P.C.Org. that their inner view of themselves is absurd or to criticize their basic feelings about loneliness and ephemerality of life. In some ways, these are the only possibilities they have of establishing a relationship with reality. The problem, therefore, is to enable them to elaborate a model of themselves in which these basic emotional schemata could also be experienced as a creative way of ordering reality and not only as an inescapable and painful existential condition.

Finally, the therapist's directiveness may, of course, be expressed by using classic behavioral and cognitive techniques. It is important to emphasize that generally the therapist employs these techniques for disproving client's superficial beliefs and expectations and in doing so allows deeper structures to emerge (see Guidano & Liotti, 1983). In this sense, a systems/process-oriented therapist does not consider the achievement of a therapeutic goal as a matter of choosing the "right" technique, but rather, he/she always uses existing techniques—or even "invents" new techniques—within the strategy of guiding the client's processes to make the tacit explicit.

REFERENCES

Aaronson, B. S. Time, time stance, and existence. In J. T. Fraser, F. C. Haber, & G. H. Muller (Eds.), *The study of time*. New York: Springer, 1972.

Abelson, R. P. Psychological status of the script concept. *American Psychologist*, 1981, *36*, 715–729.

Abramson, L. Y., Seligman, M. E. P., & Teasdale, J. D. Learned helplessness in humans: Critique and reformulation. *Journal of Abnormal Psychology*, 1978, *87*, 49–74.

Adam, K. S. Loss, suicide, and attachment. In C. M. Parkes & J. Stevenson-Hinde (Eds.), *The place of attachment in human behavior*. London: Tavistock, 1982.

Adams, P. L. *Obsessive children*. New York: Brunner/Mazel, 1973.

Ainsworth, M. D. S. Attachment as related to mother–infant interaction. *Advances in the Study of Behavior*, 1979, *9*, 2–52.

Ainsworth, M. D. S., Blehar, M. C., Waters, E., & Wall, S. *Patterns of attachment*. Hillsdale, NJ: Erlbaum, 1978.

Airenti, G., Bara, B. G., & Colombetti, M. Semantic network representation of conceptual and episodic knowledge. In R. Trappl (Ed.), *Advances in cybernetics and system research* (Vol. 11). Washington, DC: Hemisphere, 1982a.

Airenti, G., Bara, B. G., & Colombetti, M. A two level model of knowledge and belief. In R. Trappl (Ed.), *Proceedings of the Sixth European Meeting on Cybernetics and Systems Research*. Amsterdam: North-Holland, 1982b.

Allen, P. M. The evolutionary paradigm of dissipative structures. In E. R. Jantsch (Ed.), *Toward a unifying paradigm of physical, biological, and sociocultural evolution*. Boulder, CO.: Westview, 1981.

Arnkoff, D. B. Psychotherapy from the perspective of cognitive therapy. In M. J. Mahoney (Ed.), *Psychotherapy process*. New York: Plenum, 1980.

Arrindell, W. A., Emmelkamp, P. M. G., Monsma, A., & Brilman, E. The role of perceived parental practices in the aetiology of phobic disorders: A controlled study. *British Journal of Psychiatry*, 1983, *143*, 183–187.

Atlan, H. *Entre le cristal et la fumée*. Paris: Seuil, 1979.

Atlan, H. Hierarchical self-organization in living systems. In M. Zeleny (Ed.), *Autopoiesis: A theory of living organization*. New York: North-Holland, 1981.

Baltes, P. B. Life-span developmental psychology: Some converging observations on history and theory. In P. B. Baltes & O. G. Brim (Eds.), *Life-span development and behavior* (Vol. 2). New York: Academic Press, 1979.

Baltes, P. B., Reese, H. W., & Lipsitt, L. P. Life-span developmental psychology. *Annual Review of Psychology*, 1980, *31*, 65–110.

Bandura, A. *Principles of behavior modification*. New York: Holt, Rinehart & Winston, 1969.

Bandura, A. *Social foundations of thought and action: A social cognitive theory*. Englewood Cliffs, NJ: Prentice-Hall, 1985.

Bara, B. G. Changing connections between knowledge representation and problem solving. In M. Borillo (Ed.), *Représentation des connaissances et raisonnement dans les sciences de l'homme et de la société*. Le Chesnay: Editions Inria-CNRS, 1980.

Bara, B. G. Modifications of knowledge by memory processes. In M. A. Reda & M. J. Mahoney (Eds.), *Cognitive psychotherapies*. Cambridge, MA: Ballinger, 1984.

Barnett, J. On cognitive disorders in the obsessional. *Contemporary Psychoanalysis*, 1966, *2*, 122–134.

Bartlett, F. C. *Remembering*. Cambridge: Cambridge University Press, 1932.

Bateson, G., Jackson, D. D., Haley, J., & Weakland, J. Toward a theory of schizophrenia. *Behavioral Science*, 1956, *1*, 251–264.

Beardslee, W. R., Bemporad, J., Keller, M. B., & Klerman, G. L. Children of parents with major affective disorders: A review. *American Journal of Psychiatry*, 1983, *140*, 825–832.

Beattie-Emery, O., & Csikszentmihalyi, M. An epistemological approach to psychiatry: On the psychology/psychopathology of knowledge. *Journal of Mind and Behavior*, 1981, *2*, 375–396.

Beck, A. T. *Depression: Clinical, experimental, and theoretical aspects*. New York: Harper & Row, 1967.

Beck, A. T. *Cognitive therapy and the emotional disorders*. New York: International Universities Press, 1976.

Beck, A. T., Rush, A. J., Shaw, B. F., & Emery, G. *Cognitive therapy of depression*. New York: Guilford, 1979.

Beech, H. R. (Ed.). *Obsessional states*. London: Methuen, 1974.

Berg, I., Butler, A., & Hall, G. The outcome of adolescent school phobia. *British Journal of Psychiatry*, 1976, *128*, 80–85.

Berg, I., Marks, I., McGuire, R., & Lipsedge, M. School phobia and agoraphobia. *Psychological Medicine*, 1974, *4*, 428–434.

Berger, P. L., & Luckmann, T. *The social construction of reality*. Garden City, NY: Doubleday, 1966.

Bernstein, R. M. The development of the self-system during adolescence. *Journal of Genetic Psychology*, 1980, *136*, 231–245.

Bertenthal, B. I., & Fischer, K. W. Development of self-recognition in the infant. *Developmental Psychology*, 1978, *14*, 44–50.

Bever, T. G., Fodor, J. A., & Garrett, M. A formal limitation of associationism. In T. R. Dixon & D. L. Horton (Eds.), *Verbal behavior and general behavior theory*. Englewood Cliffs, NJ: Prentice-Hall, 1968.

Bickhard, M. H. A model of developmental and psychological processes. *Genetic Psychology Monographs*, 1980, *102*, 61–116.

Biller, H. B. *Paternal deprivation*. Lexington, MA: Lexington Books/D.C. Heath, 1974.

Black, A. The natural history of obsessional neurosis. In H. R. Beech (Ed.), *Obsessional states*. London: Methuen, 1974.

Blanco, S., & Reda, M. A. *Personal cognitive organizations and patterns of psychophysiological responses*. Paper presented at the Second National Convention of the Italian Society of Behavioral and Cognitive Therapy, Florence, October 1984.

Bloom, M. V. *Adolescent–parental separation*. New York: Gardner Press, 1980.

Bower, C. Mood and memory. *American Psychologist*, 1981, *36*, 129–148.

Bower, G. H., & Gilligan, S. G. Remembering information related to one's self. *Journal of Research in Personality*, 1979, *13*, 420–432.

Bowlby, J. Process of mourning. *International Journal of Psychoanalysis*, 1961, *42*, 317–340.

Bowlby, J. *Attachment and loss* (Vol. 1: *Attachment*). New York: Basic Books, 1969.

Bowlby, J. *Attachment and loss* (Vol. 2: *Separation: Anxiety and anger*). New York: Basic Books, 1973.

Bowlby, J. The making and breaking of affectional bonds: I. Etiology and psychopathology in the light of attachment theory. *British Journal of Psychiatry*, 1977a, *130*, 201–210.

Bowlby, J. The making and breaking of affectional bonds: II. Some principles of psychotherapy. *British Journal of Psychiatry*, 1977b, *130*, 421–431.

Bowlby, J. On knowing what you are not supposed to know and feeling what you are not supposed to feel. *Canadian Journal of Psychiatry*, 1979, *24*, 403–408.

Bowlby, J. *Attachment and loss* (Vol. 3: *Loss, sadness and depression*). London: Hogarth Press, 1980a.

Bowlby, J. *Caring for young: Some influences on its development*. Paper presented at the Conference on Parenthood as an Adult Experience, Michael Reese Hospital, Chicago, March 1980b.

Bowlby, J. *Attachment and loss* (Vol. 1: *Attachment*) (2nd ed.). London: Hogarth Press, 1983.

Bowlby, J. The role of childhood experience in cognitive disturbance. In M. J. Mahoney & A. Freeman (Eds.), *Cognition and psychotherapy*. New York: Plenum, 1985.

Bransford, J. D., McCarrell, N. S., Franks, J. J., & Nitsch, K. E. Toward unexplaining memory. In R. Shaw & J. D. Bransford (Eds.), *Perceiving, acting, and knowing*. Hillsdale, NJ: Erlbaum, 1977.

Brazelton, T. B. *Toddlers and parents*. Harmondsworth: Penguin Books, 1974.

Brazelton, T. B. Precursors for the development of emotions in early infancy. In R. Plutchik & H. Kellerman (Eds.), *Emotion: Theory, research, and experience* (Vol. 2). New York: Academic Press, 1983.

Brazelton, T. B., Koslowski, B., & Main, M. The origins of reciprocity: The early mother–infant interaction. In M. Lewis & L. A. Rosenblum (Eds.), *The effect of the infant on its caregiver*. New York: Wiley, 1974.

Brent, S. B. Individual specialization, collective adaptation, and rate of environmental change. *Human Development*, 1978a, *21*, 21–33.

Brent, S. B. Prigogine's model for self-organization in nonequilibrium systems:

Its relevance for developmental psychology. *Human Development*, 1978b, *21*, 374–387.

Brent, S. B. *Psychological and social structures*. Hillsdale, NJ: Erlbaum, 1984.

Bronowski, J. *The identity of man*. Garden City, NY: American Museum Science Books, 1971.

Bronowski, J., & Bellugi, U. Language, name, and concept. *Science*, 1970, *168*, 669–673.

Broughton, J. M. The divided self in adolescence. *Human Development*, 1981, *24*, 13–32.

Broughton, J. M., & Riegel, K. F. Developmental psychology and the self. *Annals of the New York Academy of Sciences*, 1977, *291*, 149–167.

Brown, G. W. Early loss and depression. In C. M. Parkes & J. Stevenson-Hinde (Eds.), *The place of attachment in human behavior*. London: Tavistock, 1982.

Brown, G. W., & Harris, T. *Social origins of depression*. London: Tavistock, 1978.

Bruch, H. *Eating disorders: Obesity, anorexia nervosa and the person within*. New York: Basic Books, 1973.

Bruch, H. *The golden cage: The enigma of anorexia nervosa*. New York: Vintage Books, 1978.

Bruch, H. Preconditions for the development of anorexia nervosa. *American Journal of Psychoanalysis*, 1980, *40*, 169–172.

Bugental, J. F. T. *Psychotherapy and process*. Reading, MA: Addison-Wesley, 1978.

Bugental, J. F. T., & Bugental, E. A fate worse than death: The fear of changing. *Psychotherapy*, 1984, *21*, 543–549.

Cacioppo, J. T., & Petty, R. E. Electromyograms as measures of extent and affectivity of information processing. *American Psychologist*, 1981, *36*, 441–456.

Campbell, D. T. Evolutionary epistemology. In P. A. Schilpp (Ed.), *The philosophy of Karl Popper*. La Salle, IL: Library of Living Philosophers, 1974.

Chandler, M. J. Relativism and the problem of epistemological loneliness. *Human Development*, 1975, *18*, 171–180.

Charlesworth, W. R. The role of surprise in cognitive development. In D. Elkind & J. Flavell (Eds.), *Studies in cognitive development*. London and New York: Oxford University Press, 1969.

Charlesworth, W. R. Human intelligence as adaptation: An ethological approach. In L. B. Resnick (Ed.), *The nature of intelligence*. Hillsdale, NJ: Erlbaum, 1976.

Churchland, P. M. *Matter and consciousness. A contemporary introduction to the philosophy of mind*. Cambridge, MA: MIT Press/Bradford Books, 1984.

Cioran, E. M. *La tentation d'exister*. Paris: Gallimard, 1956.

Cioran, E. M. *Ecartèlement*. Paris: Gallimard, 1979.

Clark, R. W. *Einstein: The life and times*. New York: McGraw-Hill, 1971.

Coleman, R. E. Cognitive–behavioral treatment of agoraphobia. In G. Emery, S. D. Hollon, & R. C. Bedrosian (Eds.), *New directions in cognitive therapy*. New York: Guilford, 1981.

Collins, A. M., & Loftus, E. F. A spreading–activation theory of semantic processing. *Psychological Review*, 1975, *82*, 407–428.

Cooley, C. H. *Human nature and the social order*. New York: Scribner, 1902.

Cooper, S. F., Leach, C., Storer, D., & Tonge, W. L. The children of psychiatric patients. *British Journal of Psychiatry*, 1977, *131*, 514–522.

Crandall, V. C., & Crandall, B. W. Maternal and childhood behaviors as antecedents of internal–external control perceptions in young adulthood. In H. M. Lefcourt (Ed.), *Research with the locus of control construct* (Vol. 2: *Developments and social problems*). New York: Academic Press, 1983.

Crase, S. J., Foss, C. J., & Colbert, K. K. Children's self-concept and perception of parents' behavior. *Journal of Psychology*, 1981, *108*, 297–303.

Csikszentmihalyi, M., & Beattie, O. V. Life themes: A theoretical and empirical exploration of their origins and effects. *Journal of Humanistic Psychology*, 1979, *19*, 45–63.

Csikszentmihalyi, M., & Rochberg-Halton, E. *The meaning of things. Domestic symbols and the self.* Cambridge: Cambridge University Press, 1981.

Davidson, R. J. Consciousness and information processing: A biocognitive perspective. In J. M. Davidson & R. J. Davidson (Eds.), *The psychobiology of consciousness.* New York: Plenum, 1980.

Dell, P. F. Beyond homeostasis: Toward a concept of coherence. *Family Process*, 1982, *21*, 21–41.

Dell, P. F., & Goolishian, H. A. "Order through fluctuation": An evolutionary epistemology for human systems. *Australian Journal of Family Therapy*, 1981, *2*, 175–184.

DeLozier, P. P. Attachment theory and child abuse. In C. M. Parkes & J. Stevenson-Hinde (Eds.), *The place of attachment in human behavior.* London: Tavistock, 1982.

Dennett, D. *Brainstorms.* Montgomery, VT: Bradford Books, 1978.

Dickstein, E. B. Self and self-esteem: Theoretical foundations and their implications for research. *Human Development*, 1977, *20*, 129–140.

Dickstein, E. B., & Posner, J. M. Self-esteem and relationship with parents. *Journal of Genetic Psychology*, 1978, *133*, 273–276.

Diener, C. I., & Dweck, C. S. An analysis of learned helplessness: II. The processing of success. *Journal of Personality and Social Psychology*, 1980, *39*, 940–952.

Dobson, K. S. (Ed.). *Handbook of cognitive–behavioral therapies.* New York: Guilford, in press.

Eibl-Eibesfeldt, I. *Love and hate. The natural history of behavior patterns.* New York: Holt, Rinehart & Winston, 1972.

Eibl-Eibesfeldt, I. Ritual and ritualization from a biological perspective. In M. von Cranach, K. Foppa, W. Lepenies, & D. Ploog (Eds.), *Human ethology.* Cambridge: Cambridge University Press, 1979.

Ekman, P. Universal and cultural differences in facial expression of emotion. In J. K. Cole (Ed.), *Nebraska symposium on motivation, 1971.* Lincoln: University of Nebraska Press, 1972.

Ellis, A. *Reason and emotion in psychotherapy.* New York: Stuart, 1962.

Emmelkamp, P. M. G. *Phobic and obsessive disorders: Theory, research, and practice.* New York: Plenum, 1982.

Epstein, S. The self-concept revisited: Or a theory of a theory. *American Psychologist*, 1973, *28*, 404–416.

Ericsson, K. A., & Simon, H. A. Verbal reports as data. *Psychological Review*, 1980, *87*, 215–251.

Erikson, E. H. *Childhood and society.* New York: Norton, 1963.

Flavell, J. H. *Cognitive development*. Englewood Cliffs, NJ: Prentice-Hall, 1977.

Flavell, J. H. Metacognitive development. In J. M. Scandura & C. J. Brainerd (Eds.), *Structural/process models of complex human behavior*. The Netherlands: Sijthoff & Noordhoff, 1978.

Flavell, J. H. Metacognition and cognitive monitoring. *American Psychologist*, 1979, 34, 906–911.

Forman, G. E. *Action and thought: From sensorimotor schemes to symbolic operations*. New York: Academic Press, 1982.

Franks, J. J. Toward understanding understanding. In W. B. Weimer & D. S. Palermo (Eds.), *Cognition and the symbolic processes*. Hillsdale, NJ: Erlbaum, 1974.

Gabor, D. Holography, 1948–1971. *Science*, 1972, 177, 299–313.

Gallup, G. G. Chimpanzees: Self-recognition. *Science*, 1970, 167, 86–87.

Gallup, G. G. Self-recognition in primates. *American Psychologist*, 1977, 32, 329–338.

Gallup, G. G., & McClure, M. K. Preference for mirror-image stimulation in differentially reared rhesus monkeys. *Journal of Comparative and Physiological Psychology*, 1971, 75, 403–407.

Gallup, G. G., McClure, M. K., Hill, S. D., & Bundy, R. A. Capacity for self-recognition in differentially reared chimpanzees. *Psychological Record*, 1971, 21, 69–74.

Gazzaniga, M. S., & LeDoux, J. E. *The integrated mind*. New York: Plenum, 1978.

Gelman, R. Preschool thought. *American Psychologist*, 1979, 34, 900–905.

Giblin, P. T. Affective development in children: An equilibrium model. *Genetic Psychology Monographs*, 1981, 103, 3–30.

Gittleson, N. L. The effect of obsessions in depressive psychosis. *British Journal of Psychiatry*, 1966a, 112, 253–259.

Gittleson, N. L. The phenomenology of obsessions in depressive psychosis. *British Journal of Psychiatry*, 1966b, 112, 261–264.

Gittleson, N. L. The fate of obsessions in depressive psychosis. *British Journal of Psychiatry*, 1966c, 112, 705–708.

Gittleson, N. L. Dpressive psychosis in the obsessional neurotic. *British Journal of Psychiatry*, 1966d, 112, 883–887.

Goldfried, M. R. (Ed.). *Converging themes in psychotherapy*. New York: Springer, 1982.

Gould, R. L. *Transformations: Growth and change in adult life*. New York: Simon & Schuster, 1978.

Gould, S. J. *Ontogeny and phylogeny*. Cambridge, MA: Harvard University Press, 1977.

Gould, S. J. *The panda's thumb: More reflections in natural history*. New York: Norton, 1980.

Greenberg, L. S. A task analysis of intrapersonal conflict resolution. In L. N. Rice & L. S. Greenberg (Eds.), *Patterns of change: Intensive analysis of psychotherapy process*. New York: Guilford, 1984.

Greenberg, L. S., & Safran, J. D. Integrating affect and cognition: A perspective on the process of therapeutic change. *Cognitive Therapy and Research*, 1984, 8, 559–578.

Greenwald, A. G. The totalitarian ego: Fabrication and revision of personal history. *American Psychologist*, 1980, 35, 603–618.

Guidano, V. F. A constructivistic outline of cognitive processes. In M. A. Reda & M. J. Mahoney (Eds.), *Cognitive psychotherapies*. Cambridge, MA: Ballinger, 1984.

Guidano, V. F. A systems, process-oriented approach to cognitive therapy. In K. S. Dobson (Ed.), *Handbook of cognitive–behavioral therapies*. New York: Guilford, in press.

Guidano, V. F., & Liotti, G. *Cognitive processes and emotional disorders*. New York: Guilford, 1983.

Guidano, V. F., & Liotti, G. A constructivistic foundation for cognitive therapy. In M. J. Mahoney & A. Freeman (Eds.), *Cognition and psychotherapy*. New York: Plenum, 1985.

Gur, R. C., & Sackeim, H. A. Self-deception: A concept in search of a phenomenon. *Journal of Personality and Social Psychology*, 1979, 37, 147–169.

Halwes, T., & Wire, B. A possible solution to the pattern recognition problem in the speech modality. In W. B. Weimer & D. S. Palermo (Eds.), *Cognition and the symbolic processes*. Hillsdale, NJ: Erlbaum, 1974.

Hamlyn, D. Person perception and our understanding of others. In T. Mischel (Ed.), *Understanding other persons*. Totowa, NJ: Rowman & Littlefield, 1974.

Hamlyn, D. Self-knowledge. In T. Mischel (Ed.), *The self: Psychological and philosophical issues*. Oxford: Basil Blackwell, 1977.

Harlow, H. F., The nature of love. *American Psychologist*, 1958, 13, 673–685.

Harlow, H. F., & Harlow, M. K. The affectional system. In A. M. Schrier, H. F. Harlow, & F. Stollnitz (Eds.), *Behavior of nonhuman primates* (Vol. 2). New York: Academic Press, 1965.

Harlow, H. F., Joslyn, D., Senko, M., & Dopp, A. Behavioral aspects of reproduction in primates. *Journal of Animal Science*, 1966, 25, 49–67.

Haviland, J. M. Personality development from childhood to young adulthood: Thinking, feeling, and self in Woolf's writing. In C. E. Izard, J. Kagan, & R. Zajonc (Eds.), *Emotions, cognitions, and behavior*. New York: Cambridge University Press, 1983.

Hawkins, R. C. *Cognitive processes in bulimia*. Paper presented at the Special Interest Group Meeting on Obesity and Eating Disorders, Association for Advancement of Behavior Therapy, Washington, DC, December 1983.

Hayek, F. A. *The sensory order*. Chicago: University of Chicago Press, 1952.

Hayek, F. A. *New studies in philosophy, politics, economics, and the history of ideas*. Chicago: University of Chicago Press, 1978.

Hayes, K. J., & Nissen, C. H. Higher mental functions in a home-raised chimpanzee. In A. M. Schrier & F. Stollnitz (Eds.), *Behavior of nonhuman primates* (Vol. 3). New York: Academic Press, 1971.

Henderson, S. The significance of social relationships in the etiology of neurosis. In C. M. Parkes & J. Stevenson-Hinde (Eds.), *The place of attachment in human behavior*. London: Tavistock, 1982.

Henderson, S., Byrne, D. G., & Duncan-Jones, P. *Neurosis and the social environment*. New York: Academic Press, 1981.

Hennessy, J. W., Kaplan, J. N., Mendoza, S. P., Lowe, E. L., & Levine, S. Separation distress and attachment in surrogate-reared squirrel monkeys. *Physiology and Behavior*, 1979, 23, 1017–1023.

Hetherington, E. M. Effects of father-absence on personality development in adolescent daughters. *Developmental Psychology*, 1972, 7, 313–326.

Hetherington, E. M., & Parke, R. D. *Child psychology: A contemporary viewpoint.* New York: McGraw-Hill, 1979.

Hinde, R. A. *Toward understanding relationships.* London: Academic Press, 1979.

Hoffman, M. L. Identification and conscience development. *Child Development*, 1971, 42, 1071–1082.

Hoffman, M. L. Developmental synthesis of affect and cognition and its implications for altruistic motivation. *Developmental Psychology*, 1975, 11, 607–622.

Hoffman, M. L. Toward a theory of empathic arousal and development. In M. Lewis & L. A. Rosenblum (Eds.), *The development of affect.* New York: Plenum, 1978.

Hunt, J. McV. Psychological development: Early experience. *Annual Review of Psychology*, 1979, 30, 103–143.

Izard, C. E. *Human emotions.* New York: Plenum, 1977.

Izard, C. E. The emergence of emotions and the development of consciousness in infancy. In J. M. Davidson & R. J. Davidson (Eds.), *The psychobiology of consciousness.* New York: Plenum, 1980.

Izard, C. E., & Buechler, S. Aspects of consciousness and personality in terms of differential emotions theory. In R. Plutchik & H. Kellerman (Eds.), *Emotion: Theory, research, and experience* (Vol. 1). New York: Academic Press, 1980.

Izard, C. E., & Buechler, S. On the emergence, functions, and regulation of some emotion expressions in infancy. In R. Plutchik & H. Kellerman (Eds.), *Emotion: Theory, research, and experience* (Vol. 2). New York: Academic Press, 1983.

Jacobson, E. The electrophysiology of mental activities. *American Journal of Psychology*, 1932, 44, 677–694.

Jantsch, E. *The self-organizing universe.* New York: Pergamon, 1980.

Jantsch, E., & Waddington, C. H. (Eds.). *Evolution and consciousness: Human systems in transition.* Reading, MA: Addison-Wesley, 1976.

Jayaratne, S. Child abusers as parents and children: A review. *Social Work*, 1977, 22, 5–9.

Johnson-Laird, P. N. *Mental models: Toward a cognitive science of language, inference, and consciousness.* Cambridge, MA: Harvard University Press, 1984.

Johnson-Laird, P. N., & Bara, B. G. Syllogistic inference. *Cognition*, 1984, 16, 1–61.

Kramer, J. R. *Family interfaces: Transgenerational patterns.* New York: Brunner/Mazel, 1985.

Kuhn, T. S. *The structure of scientific revolutions* (rev. ed.). Chicago: University of Chicago Press, 1970.

Kuhn, T. S. *The essential tension.* Chicago: University of Chicago Press, 1977.

Lakatos, I. Falsification and the methodology of scientific research programs. In I. Lakatos & A. Musgrave (Eds.), *Criticism and the growth of knowledge.* London: Cambridge University Press, 1974.

Lamb, M. E. (Ed.). *The role of the father in child development.* New York: Wiley, 1976.

Lang, P. J. A bio-informational theory of emotional imagery. *Psychophysiology*, 1979, 16, 495–512.

Langer, J. Logic in infancy. *Cognition*, 1981, *10*, 181–186.

Langer, J. From prerepresentational to representational cognition. In G. E. Forman (Ed.), *Action and thought*. New York: Academic Press, 1982.

Laszlo, E. *Introduction to systems philosophy: Toward a new paradigm of contemporary thought*. New York: Gordon & Breach, 1972.

Laszlo, E. *Systems science and world order*. Oxford: Pergamon, 1983.

Laughlin, H. P. *The neuroses*. London: Butterworths, 1967.

Leahy, R. L. Parental practices and the development of moral judgment and self-image disparity during adolescence. *Developmental Psychology*, 1981, *17*, 580–594.

Lerner, R. M., & Busch-Rossnagel, N. A. (Eds.), *Individuals as producers of their development: A life-span perspective*. New York: Academic Press, 1981.

Lerner, R. M., Skinner, E. A., & Sorell, G. T. Methodological implications of contextual/dialectic theories of development. *Human Development*, 1980, *23*, 225–235.

Leventhal, H. A perceptual–motor processing model of emotion. In P. Pliner, K. R. Blankstein, & I. M. Spigel (Eds.), *Perceptions of emotions in self and others*. New York: Plenum, 1979.

Leventhal, H. Toward a comprehensive theory of emotion. In L. Berkowitz (Ed.), *Advances in experimental social psychology* (Vol. 13). New York: Academic Press, 1980.

Levine, S. Comparative and psychobiological perspectives on development. In W. A. Collins (Ed.), *The concept of development*. Hillsdale, NJ: Erlbaum, 1982.

Levinson, D. J. The psychosocial development of men in early adulthood and the mid-life transition. In M. Roff & D. F. Ricks (Eds.), *Life history research in psychopathology*. Minneapolis: University of Minnesota Press, 1970.

Levinson, D. J. *The seasons of a man's life*. New York: Knopf, 1978.

Lewis, M., & Brooks-Gunn, J. *Social cognition and the acquisition of self*. New York: Plenum, 1979.

Lewis, M., & Rosenblum, L. A. (Eds.). *The effect of the infant on its caregiver*. New York: Wiley, 1974.

Lewis, M., & Weinraub, M. The father's role in the child's social network. In M. E. Lamb (Ed.), *The role of the father in child development*. New York: Wiley, 1976.

Linden, E. *Apes, men, and language*. New York: Penguin, 1974.

Liotti, G. Cognitive therapy, attachment theory, and psychiatric nosology. In M. A. Reda & M. J. Mahoney (Eds.), *Cognitive psychotherapies*. Cambridge, MA: Ballinger, 1984.

Liotti, G., & Guidano, V. F. Behavioral analysis of marital interaction in agoraphobic male patients. *Behaviour Research and Therapy*, 1976, *14*, 161–162.

Liotti, G., & Reda, M. A. Some epistemological remarks on cognitive therapy, behavior therapy, and psychoanalysis. *Cognitive Therapy and Research*, 1981, *5*, 231–236.

Lorenz, K. *Die ruckseite des spiegels*. Munich: Piper, 1973. (English translation, *Behind the mirror*. New York: Harcourt Brace Jovanovich, 1977.)

Luckmann, T. Personal identity as an evolutionary and historical problem. In M. von Cranach, K. Foppa, W. Lepenies, & D. Ploog (Eds.), *Human ethology*. Cambridge: Cambridge University Press, 1979.

Luria, A. R. *The nature of human conflicts: Or emotion, conflict, and will.* New York: Liveright, 1976.

Lynn, D. B. *The father: His role in child development.* Monterey, CA: Brooks/Cole, 1974.

Mahoney, M. J. *Cognition and behavior modification.* Cambridge, MA: Ballinger, 1974.

Mahoney, M. J. Psychotherapy and the structure of personal revolutions. In M. J. Mahoney (Ed.), *Psychotherapy process.* New York: Plenum, 1980.

Mahoney, M. J. Psychotherapy and human change processes. In J. H. Harvey & M. M. Parks (Eds.), *The master lecture series: Psychotherapy research and behavior change* (Vol. 1). Washington, DC: American Psychological Association, 1982.

Mahoney, M. J. Psychoanalysis and behaviorism: The yin and yang of determinism. In H. Arkowitz & S. Messer (Eds.), *Psychoanalytic and behavior therapy: Is integration possible?* New York: Plenum, 1984.

Mahoney, M. J. *Personal change processes: Notes on the facilitation of human development.* New York: Basic Books, in press.

Mahoney, M. J., & DeMonbruen, B. G. Psychology of the scientist: An analysis of problem-solving bias. *Cognitive Therapy and Research,* 1977, *1,* 229–238.

Main, M., & Weston, D. R. The quality of the toddler's relationship to mother and father: Related to conflict behavior and the readiness to establish new relationships. *Child Development,* 1981, *52,* 932–940.

Main, M., & Weston, D. R. Avoidance of the attachment figure in infancy: Descriptions and interpretations. In C. M. Parkes & J. Stevenson-Hinde (Eds.), *The place of attachment in human behavior.* London: Tavistock, 1982.

Makhlouf-Norris, F., Gwynne Jones, H., & Norris, H. Articulation of the conceptual structure in obsessional neurosis. *British Journal of Social and Cultural Psychology,* 1970, *9,* 264–274.

Makhlouf-Norris, F., & Norris, H. The obsessive–compulsive syndrome as a neurotic device for the reduction of self-uncertainty. *British Journal of Psychiatry,* 1972, *121,* 277–288.

Malatesta, C. Z., & Clayton Culver, L. Thematic and affective content in the lives of adult women: Patterns of change and continuity. In C. Z. Malatesta & C. E. Izard (Eds.), *Emotion in adult development.* Beverly Hills, CA: Sage, 1984.

Mancuso, J. C., & Ceely, S. G. The self as memory processing. *Cognitive Therapy and Research,* 1980, *4,* 1–25.

Marks, C. E. *Commissurotomy, consciousness, and unity of mind.* Montgomery, VT: Bradford Books, 1980.

Marks, I. M. *Fears and phobias.* London: Academic Press, 1969.

Markus, H. Self-schemata and processing information about the self. *Journal of Personality and Social Psychology,* 1977, *35,* 63–78.

Markus, H., & Nurius, P. Possible selves. *American Psychologist,* 1986, *41,* 954–969.

Marmor, J. Systems thinking in psychiatry: Some theoretical and clinical implications. *American Journal of Psychiatry,* 1983, *140,* 833–838.

Marris, P. Attachment and society. In C. M. Parkes & J. Stevenson-Hinde (Eds.), *The place of attachment in human behavior.* London: Tavistock, 1982.

Marshall, G. D., & Zimbardo, P. G. Affective consequences of inadequately explained physiological arousal. *Journal of Personality and Social Psychology*, 1979, *6*, 970–988.

Maslach, C. Negative emotional biasing of unexplained arousal. *Journal of Personality and Social Psychology*, 1979, *6*, 953–969.

Mathews, A. M., Gelder, M. G., & Johnston, D. W. *Agoraphobia: Nature and treatment*. New York: Guilford, 1981.

Max, L. W. An experimental study of the motor theory of consciousness: IV. Action-current responses in the deaf during awakening, kinesthetic imagery, and abstract thinking. *Journal of Comparative Psychology*, 1937, *24*, 301–344.

McGuigan, F. J. Covert oral behavior during the silent performance of language tasks. *Psychological Bulletin*, 1970, *74*, 309–326.

Mead, G. H. *Mind, self, and society*. Chicago: University of Chicago Press, 1934.

Meichenbaum, D. *Cognitive-behavior modification*. New York: Plenum, 1977.

Merikangas, K. R., Leckman, J. F., Prusoff, B. A., Pauls, D. L., & Weissman, M. M. Familial transmission of depression and alcoholism. *Archives of General Psychiatry*, 1985, *42*, 367–372.

Miller, A. Conceptual systems theory: A critical review. *Genetic Psychology Monographs*, 1978, *97*, 77–126.

Miller, A., & Wilson, P. Cognitive differentiation and integration: A conceptual analysis. *Genetic Psychology Monographs*, 1979, *99*, 3–40.

Miller, G. A. Trend and debates in cognitive psychology. *Cognition*, 1981, *10*, 215–225.

Miller, G. A., Galanter, E., & Pribram, K. H. *Plans and the structure of behavior*. New York: Holt, Rinehart & Winston, 1960.

Minuchin, S. *Families and family therapy*. Cambridge, MA: Harvard University Press, 1974.

Minuchin, S., Rosman, B. L., & Baker, L. *Psychosomatic families: Anorexia nervosa in context*. Cambridge, MA: Harvard University Press, 1978.

Money, J., & Ehrhardt, A. *Man and women, boy and girl: The differentiation and dimorphism of gender identity from conception to maturity*. Baltimore: Johns Hopkins University Press, 1972.

Montemayor, R., & Eisen, M. The development of self-conceptions from childhood to adolescence. *Developmental Psychology*, 1977, *13*, 314–319.

Morin, E. *La méthode* (Vol.1: *La nature de la nature*). Paris: Seuil, 1977.

Morin, E. Self and autos. In M. Zeleny (Ed.), *Autopoiesis: A theory of living organization*. New York: North-Holland, 1981.

Musil, R. *The man without qualities* (Vol. 1, rev. ed.). London: Pan Books, 1979.

Nagel, T. Brain bisection and the unity of consciousness. *Synthese*, 1971, *22*, 396–413.

Nagel, T. *Mortal questions*. Cambridge: Cambridge University Press, 1979.

Nakamura, R. K., & Gazzaniga, M. S. Hemispherectomy versus commissurotomy in the monkey: One hemisphere can be better than two. *Experimental Neurology*, 1978, *59*, 202–208.

Nicolis, G., & Prigogine, I. *Self-organization in nonequilibrium systems. From dissipative structures to order through fluctuations*. New York: Wiley, 1977.

Nisbett, R. E., & Wilson, T. D. Telling more than we can know: Verbal reports on mental processes. *Psychological Review*, 1977, *84*, 231–259.

Nozick, R. *Philosophical explanations*. Oxford: Clarendon Press, 1981.

Ounsted, C., Oppenheimer, R., & Lindsay, J. The psychopathology and psychotherapy of the families: Aspects of bonding failure. In A. White (Ed.), *Concerning child abuse*. Edinburgh: Churchill Livingstone, 1975.

Panksepp, J., Herman, B., Connor, R., Bishop, P., & Scott, J. P. The biology of social attachments: Opiates alleviate separation distress. *Biological Psychiatry*, 1978, *13*, 607–618.

Parker, G. Reported parental characteristics of agoraphobics and social phobics. *British Journal of Psychiatry*, 1979, *135*, 555–560.

Parker, G. Parental "affectionless control" as an antecedent to adult depression. *Archives of General Psychiatry*, 1983a, *40*, 956–960.

Parker, G. *Parental overprotection: A risk factor in psychosocial development*. London: Grune & Stratton, 1983b.

Parkes, C. M. *Bereavement: Studies of grief in adult life*. London: Tavistock, 1972.

Parkes, C. M. Attachment and the prevention of mental disorders. In C. M. Parkes & J. Stevenson-Hinde (Eds.), *The place of attachment in human behavior*. London: Tavistock, 1982.

Parkes, C. M., & Stevenson-Hinde, J. (Eds.). *The place of attachment in human behavior*. London: Tavistock, 1982.

Pask, G. Organizational closure of potentially conscious systems. In M. Zeleny (Ed.), *Autopoiesis: A theory of living organization*. New York: North-Holland, 1981.

Passingham, R. *The human primate*. San Francisco: Freeman, 1982.

Pattee, H. H. The physical basis and origin of hierarchical control. In H. H. Pattee, (Ed.), *Hierarchy theory: The challenge of complex systems*. New York: George Braziller, 1973.

Pattee, H. H. The need for complementarity in modesl of cognitive behavior: A response to Fowler and Turvey. In W. B. Weimer & D. S. Palermo (Eds.), *Cognition an the symbolic processes* (Vol. 2). Hillsdale, NJ: Erlbaum, 1982.

Peplau, L. A., & Perlman, D. *Loneliness: A sourcebook of current theory, research, and therapy*. New York: Wiley, 1982.

Piaget, J. *L'épistémologie génétique*. Paris: Presses Universitaires de France, 1970.

Piaget, J. *Biology and knowledge*. Chicago: University of Chicago Press, 1971.

Piaget, J. Intellectual evolution from adolescence to adulthood. *Human Development*, 1972, *15*, 1–12.

Piaget, J. *La prise de conscience*. Paris: Presses Universitaires de France, 1974. (English translation, *The grasp of consciousness*. Cambridge, MA: Harvard University Press, 1976.)

Plutchik, R. A general psychoevolutionary theory of emotion. In R. Plutchik & H. Kellerman (Eds.), *Emotion: Theory, research, and experience* (Vol. 1). New York: Academic Press, 1980.

Plutchik, R. Emotions in early development: A psychoevolutionary approach. In R. Plutchik & H. Kellerman (Eds.), *Emotion: Theory, research, and experience* (Vol. 2). New York: Academic Press, 1983.

Polanyi, M. *The tacit dimension*. Garden City, NY: Doubleday, 1966.

Pope, K. S., & Singer, J. L. The waking stream of consciousness. In J. M. Davidson & R. J. Davidson (Eds.), *The psychobiology of consciousness*. New York: Plenum, 1980.

Popper, K. R. *Objective knowledge: An evolutionary approach*. Oxford: Clarendon Press, 1972.

Popper, K. R. Autobiography of Karl Popper. In P. A Schilpp (Ed.), *The philosophy of Karl Popper*. La Salle, IL: Library of Living Philosophers, 1974.

Popper, K. R. The rationality of scientific revolutions. In R. Harré (Ed.), *Problems of scientific revolutions*. Oxford: Clarendon Press, 1975.

Popper, K. R. The place of mind in nature. In R. Q. Elvee (Ed.), *Mind in nature*. San Francisco: Harper & Row, 1982.

Popper, K. R., & Eccles, J. C. *The self and its brain*. New York: Springer, 1977.

Posner, M. I., & Snyder, C. R. R. Facilitation and inhibition in the processing of signals. In P. M. A. Rabbitt & S. Dornic (Eds.), *Attention and performance* (Vol. 5). New York: Academic Press, 1975.

Pound, A. Attachment and maternal depression. In C. M. Parkes & J. Stevenson-Hinde (Eds.), *The place of attachment in human behavior*. London: Tavistock, 1982.

Pribram, K. H. Emotions: Steps toward a neurophysiological theory. In D. C. Glass (Ed.), *Neurophysiology and emotion*. New York: Rockefeller University/ Russell Sage Foundation, 1967.

Pribram, K. H. *Languages of the brain*. Englewood Cliffs, NJ: Prentice-Hall, 1971.

Pribram, K. H. Some comments on the nature of the perceived universe. In R. Shaw & J. D. Bransford (Eds.), *Perceiving, acting, and knowing*. Hillsdale, NJ: Erlbaum, 1977.

Pribram, K. H. Mind, brain, and consciousness: The organization of competence and conduct. In J. M. Davidson & R. J. Davidson (Eds.), *The psychobiology of consciousness*. New York: Plenum, 1980a.

Pribram, K. H. Behaviorism, phenomenology, and holism in psychology: a scientific analysis. In R. S. Valle & R. von Eckartsberg (Eds.), *The metaphors of consciousness*. New York: Plenum, 1980b.

Pribram, K. H. The biology of emotions and other feelings. In R. Plutchik & H. Kellermen (Eds.), *Emotion: Theory, research, and experience* (Vol. 1). New York: Academic Press, 1980c.

Pribram, K. H. Reflections on the place of brain in the ecology of mind. In W. B. Weimer & D. S. Palermo (Eds.), *Cognition and the symbolic processes* (Vol. 2). Hillsdale, NJ: Erlbaum, 1982a.

Pribram, K. H. What the fuss is all about. In K. Wilber (Ed.), *The holographic paradigm and other paradoxes*. Boulder, CO: Shambala, 1982b.

Pribram, K. H. The cognitive revolution and mind/brain issues. *American Psychologist*, 1986, *41*, 507–520.

Prigogine, I. Irreversibility as a symmetry-breaking process. *Nature*, 1973, *246*, 67–71.

Prigogine, I. Order through fluctuations: Self-organization and social systems. In E. Jantsch & C. H. Waddington (Eds.), *Evolution and consciousness: Human systems in transition*. Reading, MA: Addison-Wesley, 1976.

Prigogine, I. Time, structure, and fluctuations. *Science*, 1978, *201*, 777–785.

Prigogine, I. *From time to becoming: Time and complexity in the physical sciences.* San Francisco: Freeman, 1980.

Puccetti, R. The case for mental duality: Evidence from the split-brain data and other considerations. *Behavioral and Brain Sciences*, 1981, *4*, 93–123.

Pylyshyn, Z. W. What the mind's eye tells the mind's brain: A critique of mental imagery. *Psychological Bulletin*, 1973, *80*, 1–22.

Pylyshyn, Z. W. The imagery debate: Analogue media versus tacit knowledge. *Psychological Review*, 1981a, *88*, 16–45.

Pylyshyn, Z. W. Complexity and the study of artificial and human intelligence. In J. Haugeland (Ed.), *Mind design.* Montgomery, VT: Bradford Books, 1981b.

Reber, A. S., & Lewis, S. Implicit learning: An analysis of the form and structure of a body of tacit knowledge. *Cognition*, 1977, *5*, 333–361.

Reda, M. A., & Mahoney, M. J. (Eds.). *Cognitive psychotherapies.* Cambridge, MA: Ballinger, 1984.

Reed, G. F. "Under-inclusion": A characteristic of obsessional personality disorder, I–II. *British Journal of Psychiatry*, 1969, *115*, 781–790.

Rheingold, H. L., & Eckerman, C. O. The infant separates himself from his mother. *Science*, 1970, *168*, 78–83.

Riegel, K. F. The dialectics of human development. *American Psychologist*, 1976, *31*, 689–700.

Riegel, K. F. *Foundations of dialectical psychology.* New York: Academic Press, 1979.

Rogers, T. B., Kuiper, N. A., & Kirker, W. S. Self-reference and the encoding of personal information. *Journal of Personality and Social Psychology*, 1977, *35*, 677–688.

Rosen, A. C., & Rekers, G. A. Toward a taxonomic framework for variables of sex and gender. *Genetic Psychology Monographs*, 1980, *102*, 191–218.

Russell, J. M. Saying, feeling, and self-deception. *Behaviorism*, 1978, *6*, 27–43.

Rutter, M. *Maternal deprivation reassessed.* Harmondsworth: Penguin, 1972.

Rutter, M. Maternal deprivation 1972–1978: New findings, new concepts, new approaches. *Annals of the Academy of Medicine* (Singapore), 1979, *8*, 312–323.

Salzman, L. *The obsessive personality.* New York: Aronson, 1973.

Sameroff, A. J. Development and the dialectic: The need for a systems approach. In W. A. Collins (Ed.), *The concept of development.* Hillsdale, NJ: Erlbaum, 1982.

Sander, L. W. Infant and caretaking environment. In E. J. Anthony (Ed.), *Explorations in child psychiatry.* New York: Plenum, 1975.

Schaffer, H. R., & Crook, C. K. Child compliance and maternal control techniques. *Developmental Psychology*, 1980, *16*, 54–61.

Schank, R. C., & Abelson, R. P. *Scripts, plans, goals, and understanding.* Hillsdale, NJ: Erlbaum, 1977.

Seligman, M. E. P. Depression and learned helplessness. In R. J. Friedman & M. M. Katz (Eds.), *The psychology of depression: Contemporary theory and research.* New York: Wiley, 1974.

Seligman, M. E. P. *Helplessness: On depression, development, and death.* San Francisco: Freeman, 1975.

Seligman, M. E. P., Abramson, L. Y., Semmel, A., & von Baeyer, C. Depressive attributional style. *Journal of Abnormal Psychology*, 1979, *88*, 242–247.

Selvini-Palazzoli, M. P. *Self-starvation: From individual family therapy in the treatment of anorexia nervosa* (2nd ed.). New York: Aronson, 1978.

Shaw, B. F. The theoretical and experimental foundations of a cognitive model for depression. In P. Pliner, K. R. Blankstein, &·I. M. Spigel (Eds.), *Perception of emotion in self and others*. New York: Plenum, 1979.

Shaw, B. F., & Dobson, K. S. Cognitive assessment of depression. In T. V. Merluzzi, C. R. Glass, & M. Genest (Eds.), *Cognitive assessment*. New York: Guilford, 1981.

Shaw, R. E., & McIntyre, M. Algoristic foundations to cognitive psychology. In W. B. Weimer & D. S. Palermo (Eds.), *Cognition and the symbolic processes*. Hillsdale, NJ: Erlbaum, 1974.

Sheehy, G. *Passages: Predictable crises of adult life*. New York: Bantam Books, 1976.

Shevrin, H., & Dickman, S. The psychological unconscious: A necessary assumption for all psychological theory? *American Psychologist*, 1980, *35*, 421–434.

Singer, J. L. *Imagery and daydream methods in psychotherapy and behavior modification*. New York: Academic Press, 1974.

Singer, J. L., & Antrobus, J. S. Daydreaming, imaginal processes, and personality: A normative study. In P. W. Sheehan (Ed.), *The function and nature of imagery*. New York: Academic Press, 1972.

Sirota, A. D., & Schwartz, G. E. Facial muscle patterning and lateralization during elation and depressive imagery. *Journal of Abnormal Psychology*, 1982, *91*, 25–34.

Sluzki, C. E., & Veron, E. The double bind as a universal pathogenic situation. In C. E. Sluzki & D. C. Ransom (Eds.), *Double bind*. New York: Grune & Stratton, 1976.

Sperry, R. W. Some effects of disconnecting the cerebral hemispheres. *Science*, 1982, *217*, 1223–1226.

Springer, S. P., & Deutsch, G. *Left brain, right brain*. San Francisco: Freeman, 1981.

Sroufe, L. A. The coherence of individual development. *American Psychologist*, 1979, *34*, 834–841.

Steinberg, L. D. Transformations in family relations at puberty. *Developmental Psychology*, 1981, *17*, 833–840.

Steinberg, L. D., & Hill, J. P. Patterns of family interactions as a function of age, the onset of puberty, and formal thinking. *Developmental Psychology*, 1978, *14*, 683–684.

Stern, D. N. Mother and infant at play: The dyadic interaction involving facial, vocal, and gaze behaviors. In M. Lewis & L. A. Rosenblum (Eds.), *The effect of the infant on its caregiver*. New York: Wiley, 1974.

Stewart, A. J. Personality and situation in the prediction of women's life patterns. *Psychology of Women Quarterly*, 1980, *5*, 195–206.

Stewart, A. J. The course of individual adaptation to life changes. *Journal of Personality and Social Psychology*, 1982, *42*, 1100–1113.

Stewart, A. J., & Healy, J. M. Processing affective responses to life experiences: The development of the adult self. In C. Z. Malatesta & C. E. Izard (Eds.), *Emotion in adult development*. Beverly Hills, CA: Sage, 1984.

Strauss, H., & Lewin, I. A comparative study of concept formation: A conceptual analysis. *Genetic Psychology Monographs*, 1981, *103*, 169–219.

Swann, W. B., & Read, S. J. Self-verification processes: How we sustain our self-conceptions. *Journal of Experimental and Social Psychology*, 1981, *17*, 351–372.

Tart, C. T. States of consciousness and state-specific sciencess. *Science*, 1972, *176*, 1203–1210.

Tart, C. T. A systems approach to altered states of consciousness. In J. M. Davidson & R. J. Davidson (Eds.), *The psychobiology of consciousness*. New York: Plenum, 1980.

Teuber, H. L. Why two brains? In F. O. Schmitt & F. G. Worden (Eds.), *The neurosciences: Third study program*. Cambridge, MA: MIT Press, 1974.

Thom, R. *Structural stability and morphogenesis*. Reading, MA: W. A. Benjamin, 1975.

Tomkins, S. S. Script theory: Differential magnification of affects. In H. E. Howe & M. M. Page (Eds.), *Nebraska symposium on motivation* (Vol. 24). Lincoln: University of Nebraska Press, 1978.

Turner, R. M., Steketee, G., & Foa, E. Fear of criticism in washers, checkers, and phobics. *Behaviour Research and Therapy*, 1979, *17*, 79–81.

Turner, T. Piaget's structuralism. *American Anthropologist*, 1973, *75*, 351–373.

Turvey, M. T. Constructive theory, perceptual systems, and tacit knowledge. In W. B. Weimer & D. S. Palermo (Eds.), *Cognition and the symbolic processes*. Hillsdale, NJ: Erlbaum, 1974.

Vaillant, G. E. *Adaptation to life*. Boston: Little, Brown, 1977.

Van Den Berg, O., & Eelen, P. Unconscious processing and emotions. In M. A. Reda & M. J. Mahoney (Eds.), *Cognitive psychotherapies*. Cambridge, MA: Ballinger, 1984.

Varela, F. J. On observing natural systems. *CoEvolution Quarterly*, Summer 1976a.

Varela, F. J. Not one, not two. *CoEvolution Quarterly*, Fall 1976b.

Varela, F. J. *Principles of biological autonomy*. New York: North-Holland, 1979.

Varela, F. J. Describing the logic of the living. In M. Zeleny (Ed.), *Autopoiesis: A theory of living organization*. New York: North-Holland, 1981.

Varela, F. J. The creative circles: Sketches on the natural history of circularity. In P. Watzlawick (Ed.), *The invented reality*. New York: Norton, 1984.

Wachs, T. D., & Gruen, G. E. *Early experience and human development*. New York: Plenum, 1982.

Waddington, C. H. *The strategy of genes*. London: Allen & Unwin, 1957.

Waddington, C. H. *Tools for thought*. New York: Basic Books, 1977.

Wason, P. C. On the failure to eliminate hypotheses. . . . a second look. In P. N. Johnson-Laird & P. C. Wason (Eds.), *Thinking: Readings in cognitive science*. Cambridge: Cambridge University Press, 1977.

Watanabe, S. Creative time. In J. T. Fraser, F. C. Haber, & G. H. Muller (Eds.), *The study of time*. New York: Springer, 1972.

Watts, A. W. *Nature, man, and woman*. New York: Vintage Books, 1958.

Weimer, W. B. Psycholinguistics and Plato's paradoxes of the Meno. *American Psychologist*, 1973, *28*, 15–33.

Weimer, W. B. Overview of a cognitive conspiracy: Reflections on the volume. In W. B. Weimer & D. S. Palermo (Eds.), *Cognition and the symbolic processes*. Hillsdale, NJ: Erlbaum, 1974.

Weimer, W. B. The psychology of inference and expectation: Some preliminary remarks. In G. Maxwell & R. M. Anderson (Eds.), *Minnesota studies in the philosophy of science* (Vol. 6). Minneapolis: University of Minnesota Press, 1975.

Weimer, W. B. A conceptual framework for cognitive psychology: Motor theories of the mind. In R. Shaw & J. D. Bransford (Eds.), *Perceiving, acting, and knowing*. Hillsdale, NJ: Erlbaum, 1977.

Weimer, W. B. *Notes on the methodology of scientific research*. Hillsdale, NJ: Erlbaum, 1979.

Weimer, W. B. Hayek's approach to the problems of complex phenomena: An introduction to the theoretical psychology of the sensory order. In W. B. Weimer & D. S. Palermo (Eds.), *Cognition and the symbolic processes* (Vol. 2). Hillsdale, NJ: Erlbaum, 1982a.

Weimer, W. B. Ambiguity and the future of psychology: Méditations leibniziennes. In W. B. Weimer & D. S. Palermo (Eds.), *Cognition and the symbolic processes* (Vol. 2). Hillsdale, NJ: Erlbaum, 1982b.

Weimer, W. B. *Spontaneously ordered complex phenomena*. Paper prepared for Committee I of the 12th International Conference on the Unity of the Sciences, Chicago, November 1983.

Weimer, W. B. Limitations of the dispositional analysis of behavior. In J. R. Royce & L. P. Mos (Eds.), *Annals of theoretical psychology* (Vol. 1). New York: Plenum, 1984.

Weiss, E. *Agoraphobia in the light of ego psychology*. New York: Grune & Stratton, 1964.

Weiss, R. S. Attachment in adult life. In C. M. Parkes & J. Stevenson-Hinde (Eds.), *The place of attachment in human behavior*. London: Tavistock, 1982.

Welwood, J. Self-knowledge as the basis for an integrative psychology. *Journal of Transpersonal Psychology*, 1979, *11*, 23–40.

Welwood, J. The holographic paradigm and structure of experience. In K. Wilber (Ed.), *The holographic paradigm and other paradoxes*. Boulder, CO: Shambala, 1982.

Werner, H. *Comparative psychology of mental development*. New York: International Universities Press, 1948.

Werner, H. The concept of development from a comparative and organismic point of view. In D. E. Harris (Ed.), *The concept of development*. Minneapolis: University of Minnesota Press, 1957.

White, P. Limitations on verbal reports of internal events: A refutation of Nisbett and Wilson and of Bem. *Psychological Review*, 1980, *87*, 105–112.

Wolf, D. Understanding others: A longitudinal case study of the concept of independent agency. In G. E. Forman (Ed.), *Action and thought*. New York: Academic Press, 1982.

Wolpe, J. *Theme and variations: A behavior therapy casebook*. New York: Pergamon, 1976.

Zajonc, R. B. Feeling and thinking: Preferences need no inferences. *American Psychologist*, 1980, *35*, 151–175.

Zeleny, M. (Ed.). *Autopoiesis: A theory of living organization*. New York: North-Holland, 1981.

INDEX